To Julie

Love Light e Reiki
Margo Wise Owl
—x—
3-3-11.

You'll Never Make Pastry: Your Hands are Too Hot

To Reiki Master Teacher......and beyond!

Margaret Elson

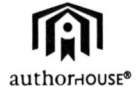

authorHOUSE®

AuthorHouse™ UK Ltd.
500 Avebury Boulevard
Central Milton Keynes, MK9 2BE
www.authorhouse.co.uk
Phone: 08001974150

© 2010 Margaret Elson. All rights reserved.

No part of this book may be reproduced, stored in a retrieval system, or transmitted by any means without the written permission of the author.

First published by AuthorHouse 4/23/2010

ISBN: 978-1-4520-1360-2 (sc)

Edited by Jan Andersen
Author of Chasing Death: Losing a Child to Suicide
http://www.creativecopywriter.org

This book is printed on acid-free paper.

I dedicate this book to the memory of my wonderful parents Harold and Henrietta Wright. I have always felt extremely lucky and fortunate to be born to these two wonderful human beings and I credit them with the person I am today. I just hope Grahame and Cheryl feel that we have gone some way to follow in my mum and dad's footsteps and that they feel truly loved and blessed with both Pip and I as their parents.

***God couldn't be everywhere,
therefore he invented mother***

- Rudyard Kipling -

Acknowledgements

To my husband "Pip", who is my rock and gives me unending support and sound advice.

To Grahame, our wonderful, sceptical son (everything has a logical explanation).

To Cheryl, our beautiful Indigo daughter, who first showed me the way of Reiki, unwittingly, and has been a constant strength and support on my Spiritual journey ever since. After having an operation on her knee, Cheryl was in a lot of discomfort and no amount of painkillers would work. I was "told" to put my hand on her knee and within seconds the pain had gone. Cheryl then told me, "You have got something there Mum; you need to learn how to use it."

The rest, as they say, is history!

To Christine Tatton, for her constant strength and support! Paul Thomas my guiding Spiritual light. To Wendy Terry, my own personal Angel and to Jan Andersen, a fellow Light Worker, who has edited my book for me!

Angela Hickman my "Angelic" guiding light. Her constant support, sound advice and help go beyond anything I could ever have wished for.

To Chris, Jackie, Rachel, Eileen and Edna for allowing me to relate their Reiki/Angel experiences!

I give humble thanks to Doreen and Collette for allowing me to use their actual names and feel privileged to mention Gwen and Jock, parents and grandparents.

Jayne Hale for her "Angelic" message prompting the writing of this book

I thank all those people that I have met as I have traversed this lifetime; without you I would not have a story to tell.

Last, but not least, to my wonderful guides who have made this book possible.

For God Himself works in our souls, in the deepest depths, taking increasing control as we are progressively willing to be prepared for His wonder.

~ Thomas R Kelly ~

Contents

Forward xi
Preface xiii
Part One: 1946-1992 1
Part Two: My Spiritual Awakening 39
Paul Thomas 41
"He's Here You Know!" 43
2002-2009: My Journey to the Present Day 45
Angela Hickman 97
Part Three: Reiki, Divine Source & The Angelic Realm 101
Reiki: A Divine Explanation 105
A History of Reiki and its Founder, Dr Mikao Usui 113
Reiki is My Life 117
Learning Non-Attachment 123
Reiki and Dying 125
Working with the "Light" 127
Explanation of the "Aura" 131
Descriptive Layers of the Aura/Human Energy Field ... 133
Colours of the Aura 137
Explanation to Chakras: Your Own Personal Energy System 141
Spheres and Colours of the Chakras 145
Explanation and Sanskrit Name of Each Individual Chakra 149
The Angelic Realm 153
An Explanation of Archangels 157
Testimonials to Belief and Believing 165
Epilogue 179
Amazing Grace 181

Foreword
By Jan Andersen

I was privileged to connect with "Mags" via a mutual friend and Light Worker, Angela Hickman, whose book (The Book of Grace/Vol I: The Lost Pages) I edited last year. Our meeting was no coincidence, since everything is about Divine timing.

It has become clear to me over the past year that many Light Workers/Earth Angels around the world are joining together in a common mission for the Higher Good, to create a "new planet Earth", built on foundations of unity and love rather than division and war. Mags is one such Earth Angel.

Editing this book was an absolute joy and honour rather than a task and I feel extremely fortunate to have been afforded a "sneak preview" of a story that I feel will offer much comfort and hope to people, not least those who are struggling to find some meaning to their lives, those enduring emotional turmoil and, of course, other emerging Earth Angels.

Chronicling her life from childhood through to the conclusion of this book, Mags takes the reader on a compelling journey via significant dates and events, emotional and physical losses and gains, angelic experiences and her spiritual awakening to Reiki Master/Teacher, Mags "Wise Owl" Elson.

I cried, laughed and had many "light bulb" moments along the way; those moments when you read about strange phenomena that you too have encountered and say, "Ah! So that explains it; it was the Angels communicating with me."

Mags shows how the Reiki experience and communicating with the Angels and the Spirit World isn't just confined to a lucky few, but is accessible to everyone, anywhere and at any time and can enrich one's life far beyond the limits of the imagination.

I won't give away too much about the book, but I feel sure that all those who read it will take something positive from it; and those who are still grappling with their faith will see the infinite possibilities when one embraces the Angels and the Reiki experience.

To be a star, you must shine your own light, follow your own path and don't worry about the darkness for that is when stars shine the brightest

- Unknown -

Preface

One minute past midnight, 5 October 1946, a Light Worker came to Earth. My name is Margaret Ann Elson and on that day I came to start my spiritual journey as a Light Worker/Earth Angel.

This is the story of my life and the journey of learning that I have undertaken on my Spiritual pathway to becoming a Reiki Master at Teacher level.

I hope this book will inspire other souls like me who, at times, have found life hard to cope with.

Without these lessons I would not be who or where I am today.

The feeling that I have had all my life of not belonging and always having to try that little bit harder to be accepted has been very hard to understand. School, workplace; you name it. I always felt different; the outsider, the onlooker standing on the periphery, wanting to be accepted and failing miserably.

The isolation I felt was very hard to cope with and to comprehend.

Becoming a Reiki Master created the feeling of "At last I have found what I have been looking for and at long last I belong".

Now I know the reason why I felt so isolated; I am a Light-worker/Earth-Angel and, of course, I could not fit in with most of mankind. How could I?

I am here to do a special job and the only way that I could connect is with my fellow Light-Workers/Earth-Angels who, like me, have come here to do our Lord's work; healing and teaching.

I know now that I worked with Jesus when he walked the Earth plane and explains why I have never ever been able to watch the Crucifixion. I was there and I was also crucified watching my Master on the cross.

"You'll never make pastry; your hands are too hot!"

These are the words that Mum constantly told me as I was growing up.

Mum was a great cook and I loved to help in the kitchen when she was baking, but unfortunately my hands were always "too hot"!

At the time, I never realised that she was giving me the title for this book!

I was born with "Reiki", the Divine gift given to Light Workers/Earth Angels and the reason why we have come back in this lifetime to finish what Jesus started.

I asked Angela Hickman, author of *The Book of Grace*, if she would graciously write the foreword for my book. Her reply to me read as follows:

"Firstly, I love the way you have written it - it is very easy to understand and I kept seeing a subtitle on it, 'If I can do it……' I realised why later.

"Rapid River came in to me as I got nearer to the end, along with Archangel Michael, Jesus and God (so if I don't tell you what they've shown me I'll get struck down with lightening!).

Rapid River showed me that all the healing stuff you do is, as yet, untapped and written. You have SO much more to offer to the world on top of this." Angela.

I now know that this book is a wakeup call to all Light Workers/Earth Angels and hopefully what I have written will resonate deep within; helping you to understand why you are here and to what your purpose is in this lifetime.

All events that I have written about in this book can be authenticated.

I substituted some details with an asterisk (*) in order to protect the identities of the people involved. This is my choice, not theirs. Some of my clients are still undergoing treatment and, as such, I felt a need to protect their privacy. Nevertheless, they are more than willing to authenticate what I have written about them should the need arise.

The spiritual quest begins, for most people, as a search for meaning

- Marilyn Ferguson -
1946 - 1957

"This is my body which is given for you.

Every time you eat bread, think of me."

"This wine is my blood that will be shed to remove the sins of all who come to believe in me and it is the start of a new agreement between God and mankind."

~ 1 Corinthians 11-24 ~

Part One:

1946-1992

Saturday 5 October 1946

On this day, at one minute past midnight, I was born to Harold and Henrietta Wright at the (then) Andressey Hospital in Burton-on-Trent, Staffordshire, England. My mum was 37-years-old and my dad was 35-years-old. I had one elder brother by the name of Derek, who was born in April 1940.

In 1942, Dad was called up to serve with the Royal Engineers as a Stevedore, working mainly in France and Belgium on the docks unloading Armed Forces' supplies.

Dad did not like to talk about the war. There were too many painful memories. One of these memories was being torpedoed whilst docked in harbour.

Dad had always been an early riser and in his own words, on that particular morning, he had "gone to the other end of the ship to have a wash and shave, when all hell broke loose". A German submarine had managed to sneak its way into the harbour and torpedoed dad's ship. This led to the loss of many young men; one of them being a young lad named "Nobby" Clark, aged 18.

The abiding memory for my dad from this incident was the sight of Nobby, with not a mark on him, floating out of the hole made by the torpedo.

This memory remained with my dad until the day he died and every year on the anniversary he remembered Nobby.

Dad came home from the war in 1945 and my birth followed in October 1946.

1953 – Aged 7

Mum was in hospital for three weeks for a Hysterectomy, which in those days was a major operation. I had three weeks of sheer misery staying at my aunt's, not caused by her, but my cousin who shall remain nameless!!

1957 – Aged 10

Mum was in hospital again for a Cholecystectomy (Gallbladder removal).

Thank goodness I was allowed to stay at home this time!

1960 – Aged 13

Mum had her left breast removed due to cancer and in those days it was referred to as a "radical mastectomy". I was blissfully unaware of the reason for Mum's operation, since cancer was not known or talked about as it is now.

Mum underwent radiotherapy treatment in the Queen Elizabeth Hospital in Birmingham and spent six horrendous weeks there, enduring this radical treatment without her family being close by to support her.

I can recall her telling us on one visit that she felt like jumping out of the window of the hospital ward. Being miles away from her family and having to suffer this gruelling treatment on her own was becoming too much!

This was extremely hard on all of us. Having no car of our own, we had to rely on Alan McMillan to take us to Birmingham, which was a good hour's car journey away from where we lived and meant that we could only go and visit twice a week.

Alan McMillan was an Earth Angel without wings. This lovely man volunteered to take us over to the Queen Elizabeth every week and all without asking and was very reluctant to take any monies that Dad offered him.

The rest of the sixties up to 1969 were spent in a blur of hospitals; Waldsgrave at Coventry, (camera down her throat), Queen Elizabeth at Birmingham (radiotherapy) and Burton Hospital, under the tender care of Mr Bond, Cancer Specialist.

1967 – July

Mum was in hospital again, this time for treatment for cancer that had now spread to the back of her eye, brain and other organs.

I have often wondered since if Mum and Dad knew the consequences of this appalling disease, because if they did, they never let on to me.

> *Mother is the name of God in the lips and hearts of children.*
>
> ~ *William Makepeace Thackeray* ~

1968 – January to August

In January of this year, Mum had double pneumonia and spent several weeks in bed at home being looked after by *Dr Shaw, a wonderful man and a true "Earth Angel".

I have always believed that it was her faith in Dr Shaw that kept her optimistic and strong in her beliefs, but even so she told him in no uncertain terms that she was stopping at home because she had had her fill of hospitals!

Our house did not have a bathroom or central heating at this time. The District Nurse used to come in and help with a bed bath and I dealt with everything else.

On 24 May, Mum finally recovered from this bout of pneumonia and it was decided that I would take her to Skegness for the May Bank holiday week, with Dad coming down on the Tuesday to spend the day with us.

We had a lovely week together, with warm weather, good "digs" and a treasured week spent in each other's company.

In June, we had only been back home a week when Mum suffered a heart attack. This was confirmed by Dr Sharkey, the Cardiac Heart Consultant from the hospital, who came to our house and performed all the necessary tests.

Both Dr Sharkey and Dr Shaw decided that Mum would fare much better at home with a District Nurse coming in to look after her, as well as myself.

Dr Shaw suggested that I ask permission for compassionate leave from work which would allow me to look after Mum at home.

At this time I was working for a local company whose manager was a *Mr Baxter

(Mr Baxter ruled with an iron fist and everyone was exceedingly nervous of him. Every time there was a full moon, the following morning he would come into work in the foulest mood possible! Strange you may say, but it was true!)

I was literally quaking in my shoes at the thought of asking him for time off, but with head held high off I went! Imagine my surprise when this blustering giant of a man got up from his seat, walked around the table, gave me a hug and said, "Margaret, you may have as long as you want off; your Mum is the most precious thing you will ever have and......I will also pay you!"

This show of emotion and action that Mr Baxter showed to me left me a blubbering idiot.

I have never felt so touched or humbled in my life before.

How wrong could you be about a person who, before this day, had never even looked at me, let alone spoken to me? Was he an Earth-Angel in disguise? I like to think so and I will be forever in his debt.

June-July - Wimbledon

Mum loved her sport. You name it, she watched it. Mum had supported Aston Villa whilst in service in Aston in the 1920s. It was really unheard of in those days; a woman going to a football match? But mum did not care; she just enjoyed watching it.

One of her greatest loves was Wimbledon, but unfortunately having suffered this heart attack meant that she could not watch it, confined to bed as she was. This was a great disappointment to her as Rod Laver was going to be playing Tony Roache in the Final.

Mum pleaded with Dr Shaw to be allowed to come downstairs and watch the final on television, (no such thing as TV in the bedroom in those days).

The laughable part of this story was Dr Shaw telling mum she could watch it providing she did not get excited...... as if!

Derek and I carried her downstairs in a chair and mum was back in pride of place watching her beloved tennis, which Rod Laver won, defeating Tony Roache in straight sets: 6-3 6-4 6-2.

I was quite disappointed in this as I was secretly in love with Tony Roache. In fact I adored him.

In my opinion, the late sixties through to the early seventies was the best time for tennis. In that era you had the most wonderful characters; Fred Stolle, John Newcombe, Roger Taylor, Jimmy Conners, Bjorn Borg and John ("You cannot be serious") McEnroe, to name but a few. Great characters and great tennis!

I was quite sad when Anne Jones won the ladies' 1969 women's tennis final beating Billie Jean King 3-6 6-3 6-2, as Mum was not around to experience this triumph for British ladies' tennis.

July-August

Due to Mum having a heart attack, my holiday to Lloret-De-Mar in Spain with my great mate Rosie (who sadly passed away in December 2000 after suffering a brain tumour at the tender age of 56) was in doubt.

I had huge reservations about going and it was not until two days before I was due to depart that Dr Shaw gave me the OK. Even so, I was still not happy about going all that way and not being at home if anything should happen to her.

I had had this fear from the age of 14 that I would lose Mum at a tender age. This abiding fear that I would not have her for long was something that I could not talk about. Who could I tell? To whom could I talk? I was haunted by death and petrified at the thought of it, without ever really understanding why.

So, Rosie and I went off to Spain; I with heavy heart and huge trepidation. I can remember, even to this day, hating every minute of the first week. However, Mum had insisted that I go and enjoy myself as it was virtually unheard of to holiday abroad - and to go on a plane? Well that's another story.

On the second Sunday, Rosie's Mum phoned to tell me that Mum was now up and about and had sent me a message not to worry, that she was fine. Even so, I could not wait to get home and see her.

In those days you had to go down to Luton Airport if you were travelling abroad, which was a nightmare. First of all you had to go to Digbeth Road Bus Station in Birmingham. For two young girls very early in the morning, it was terrifying. From there you made your way to Luton Airport.

We landed back in England in the early hours of the morning and I can remember getting home around 5.00am. I was so excited at the prospect of seeing Mum, but I was deeply disappointed. I walked into the lounge to see Dad sitting there on his own waiting to greet me when, suddenly, the door curtain was swept back and there stood Mum with her arms held out ready for me to rush into. I broke down sobbing, but at the same time I was overjoyed that she was standing there in front of me to welcome me home and to surprise me in that manner. A memory I will cherish forever.

They were good at doing surprises, Mum and Dad. I can remember when it was my twelfth birthday and we were sitting at the table having dinner. Mum asked me to pour Dad a cup of tea. My reply was "No! He can pour his own". Mum then asked me again, "Please pour your Dad a cup of tea", so reluctantly I lifted the tea cosy and there, in front of my eyes, was the most beautiful watch you had ever seen. I immediately burst into tears followed by Mum and Dad. A lovely memory!

1969

Sunday 19 January

At breakfast that morning, Mum told me that she had woken up in the night to find that she was totally pain free; not an ache or a pain anywhere. The realisation (which was to come much later) was that she was nearing "end stage" of this horrendous illness, breast cancer.

One of my abiding memories of this time was of me asking her why she had to suffer so much when there were so many awful people in the world. Her reply was, "But Jesus suffered so why shouldn't I? And, I hope that I have done the suffering for you too!" What faith! How do you answer that?

Tuesday 21 January

Late afternoon Mum went into a coma, as a result of which she did not recognise us. This was very hard to accept; heartbreaking in fact. You could speak to her and her reply would just be a repetitive, "Hello, hello".

Thursday 23 January

Mum passed away at exactly 6.00am in her own bed with Dad beside her.

Walking across the landing to their bedroom I heard the church clock striking the hour of 6.00am, followed by this strange noise coming from their bedroom. This noise was the "death rattle", which meant Mum had finally lost her battle against this most cruel disease.

Mum had gone and at long last she was free from pain, but little did we realise then our pain was only just beginning.

The next few days passed in a blur; registering the death and organising the funeral. Dad allowed me to choose cremation. The thought of my mum going in a hole in the ground filled me with dread.

It was also around this time that Dad explained to me that Mum had been battling breast cancer since the removal of her left breast in 1960. This information went straight over the top of my head. I had no comprehension whatsoever of the word "cancer" and its implications.

It was to be many years later before I realised the full extent of the suffering that mum had silently endured for so many years and all with a smile and a kind word for everyone she met. A True Earth Angel and I have always felt privileged to have had her as my mum!

Saturday 25 January

Two days later as I lay on my bed sobbing, I heard Mum's voice asking me to stop crying, telling me that she was alright now, that all her pain has gone and that she would never leave me; she would always be at my side looking over me!

I swung round expecting to see Mum standing there, but no one was there.

I sat on the side of the bed totally bemused at what I thought I had just heard, but I had definitely heard her!

I thought about going to tell Dad, because he will be so pleased to know that Mum had come back, but then a little voice told me that I couldn't because he would think I had "gone daft" and it would only upset him. So, I kept this little secret to myself, never ever telling Dad or Derek, for that matter, what had occurred in my bedroom on that fateful day!

Wednesday 29 January - Mum's funeral

At 8.30am there was a knock at the door and a small child stood there with a wreath telling me it was from the children of the street where we lived. I was too immersed in my grief to respond and even to this day could not tell you who it was. So, I turned and put it with the rest of the wreaths that were now covering the front room floor.

We were deeply shocked at the outpouring of grief from friends, neighbours and even from people that we did not know, but who had known Mum. In some small way, at this sad time, it was a comfort to know how much Mum was loved and respected by everyone, but we were too grief stricken to respond.

9.00am - High Bank Road Chapel

We walked into the Chapel which seemed to be bursting at the seams.

People had asked us to go to the Chapel first so that they could pay their respects to Mum. In those days it was difficult to get to Markeaton Crematorium on the outskirts of Derby, so we had abided by their wishes and they had not let us down.

10.30am - Markeaton Crematorium

Our journey to the crematorium was a mixture of torrential rain and high winds, but my enduring memory from this torturous journey was of looking at Mum's coffin and thinking "that thing" is now dead and can do her no more harm. This offensive thing even had the nerve to show itself outside of her body, behind her ear. Thank goodness she had not been able to see it!

We sang one of Mum's favourite hymns, "From Sinking Sands He Lifted Me" and this was the inscription we had put in the Remembrance book.

As we sat waiting for the committal to begin, the sun suddenly appeared from out of a dense and rain swept sky and shone a golden ray of sunshine directly onto her coffin. It was to be many years later before I realised the significance of this "sign". It was Mum's way of showing us that she was going "home" in a shaft of the most perfect "White Light".

Monday 17 February

After three weeks off work I felt that it was time to go back. This I was dreading. How would I cope? How would people react with me? I was filled with a constant dread at the thought of meeting and facing everyone. I was extremely worried at what my reactions were going to be and I walked into work with a heavy heart and my stomach tied up in knots.

*Gary Yeomans, who was a rather cantankerous man with whom I did not really connect, walked straight up to me, enfolded me in his arms, gave me a big hug and told me that he was so sorry that I had lost Mum. This made me crumple and I broke down in floods of tears.

To be shown such emotion from this "funny old b****r" was such a surprise and one that I will never ever forget. Was this another Earth Angel? I like to think so.

So began the dreadful business of trying to cope with life without our mainstay. The next few months passed in a blur of agony and heartache. I felt so alone, with no one to talk to, no one in whom to confide my feelings. I was totally lost and alone, drowning in my own sea of sorrow and heartache.

Dad would not let me talk of Mum; it was as if she had not existed. I know better now of course, that was the only way he could deal with losing her.

I can remember Easter of this year all too well. Dad and Derek had gone to watch Derby County play at home. I too supported Derby but I just could not face being in a crowd. Being on my own was when it really hit me. Mum had gone; she had died and left me and she would not be coming back, EVER!

I collapsed in a heap on the floor sobbing as if my heart would break. Correction; it was broken and felt like it would never, ever heal.

This woman who had nursed me through all manner of childhood ailments, starting school and starting work, Mum had always been there, offering me wisdom and support and now she had gone and left me. How on earth was I going to cope or survive?

I staggered on until the September when I broke down at a cricket match. I can vaguely remember one of the players coming up to me and saying they were deeply sorry about the loss of my mum. The next thing I can remember is being at the back of the clubhouse for what seemed hours crying as if my life depended on it and being "found" by one of the cricketers. The flood gates had opened and there was no way of stopping them.

Dad came with me the next morning to see Dr Shaw and his words to me, "I have been expecting you", are ingrained in my deepest memory.

I was diagnosed as having had a nervous breakdown, with the explanation that because of all the trauma of looking after Mum and then experiencing "nothing", this was the result.

Having no one to talk to and keeping everything bottled up inside, putting on a brave face for my dad and brother, had all taken its toll.

To say I felt suicidal at this point in my life is not an exaggeration. I did not want to live and Dr Shaw knew this and prescribed me antidepressants with the proviso that it was for a short while only.

Dad had joined the Gresley Male Voice choir in 1955 as a Top Tenor and the men of the choir were second to none in their support to Dad and his grief in losing "mother", as he always called her. This proved to be a life saver for him and gave him a reason to carry on living.

Derek had met Val in the March and they had now set up home together.

Christmas was a total non-event in our house that year. Dr Shaw had told me that after Christmas he wanted to wean me off the tablets and try to get me back to "normality". My thoughts were constantly of Mum and normality was a word that did not exist in my vocabulary.

For the next two years I struggled on as best as I could without the person who had been such a guiding influence in my life. Nevertheless, another Earth Angel was about to enter my life and help me to come to terms with my devastating loss.

***An angel is someone who helps you
believe in miracles again.***

And that is a friend, lover, or child!

- Author Unknown - 1971

In March of that year I went to work for another local company and this proved to be a life changing decision on my part. Firstly, I met Christine Tatton and it was to be where I met my future husband "Pip". I had briefly met Christine (Chris) when we both worked for the same company. Chris was in the office and I was a trainer on the shop floor.

Moving to this new place of work meant that I was in closer contact with Chris. Our friendship developed and spanned the test of time and is as strong now as it was nearly forty years ago.

Chris came into my life when I needed her most. Her sound advice and constant support have been a strength that I have recognised over the years and we would go to the ends of the earth for each other, if need be. We have laughed and cried together; more laughing than crying I hasten to add and it was through her and her Mum that indirectly helped set me on my Spiritual pathway.

Mrs Tatton took me under her wing and became a surrogate Mum to me and, just like her daughter, embraced me into the heart of their family, which included her dad and two older sisters.

Sunday 7 November

November; Three years on and still struggling to come to terms with my loss, Mrs Tatton suggested that I go to a local Spiritualist Church with her and Chris that evening. I wasn't sure about going, knowing that the purpose was to contact the dead. I knew that Dad would object if he knew that I was trying to contact Mum. Why I thought that was a mystery really, since Dad and I had never spoken of such things.

In the end, curiosity got the better of me and off we went. I was filled with trepidation at what was going to happen; this was all new to me and I had no idea what to expect. To say that I was scared is an understatement.

The first week nothing happened. I was kind of disappointed, yet at the same time relieved. The second week the medium came straight to me and told me that she had got a message for me. This scared the living daylights out of me and I didn't know what to do.

"Your Mum is standing right behind you and she is holding a bunch of yellow narcissi."

Narcissi were Mum's favourite flowers. How could she know that?

"And you have to check the bike as the wheel is loose."

What on earth was this woman going on about?

"Your Mum is asking me to tell you that she wants you to stop grieving so hard and to get on with your life. She has not left you and she is still looking over you and will never leave you. Come May blossom, all your troubles will be over."

What troubles? May Blossom, Narcissi, bike...

At that point she turned and went to someone else.

I just sat there for the rest of the service in shock, going over and over in my mind what the medium had said. How could she tell me those things? She did not even know my mum, but she had told me about the Narcissi hadn't she? And they were Mum's words when she came to me in my bedroom. She hadn't left me and she has given me a message to prove it!

That was to be my first encounter with the "other side".

I came out of that church with a totally new outlook on life. Mum was fine and she was still with me; ok, so not in the physical sense, but she was definitely with me in spirit.

Dad had a bike he had not ridden in years, but a fortnight after receiving the above message at the spiritual church, a neighbour came round and asked if he could borrow it. This brought to mind the message about the bike wheel being loose. How on earth was I going to tell Dad that!

I did not have to. "You had better give it a good overhaul before you ride it," Dad advised the neighbour. I have often wondered if those words were put into his mouth.

What did that experience teach me that day and every day since then? The majority of us need to have that contact. To be given proof that our loved ones are still around and watching over us contributes greatly towards helping us to learn to "live" with our grief.

1972

May Blossom? That too was soon to be revealed. Unbeknownst to me, I had been suffering with Gallstones for six months. I had started with bouts of the most intense pain and sickness in November of 1971, with the Doctor diagnosing me as suffering from chronic indigestion.

Over the next few months the attacks became more frequent and the intensity and duration became longer and unbearable.

On Tuesday 18 April Dad had called the doctor out as I was in so much pain, stemming from my abdomen and going round into my back; almost as if a tight belt was there, preventing me from breathing.

*Dr Davies was less than sympathetic and told me that I had to "put up" with it as there was nothing else he could do other than keep prescribing me indigestion medicine.

On Sunday 23 April at 3pm, the pain suddenly increased in its intensity. It was so excruciating that I felt I was going to die!

"Please let me call the doctor," was Dad's constant plea throughout the afternoon and into the early night.

I had felt such a fool on the Tuesday when Dr Davies told me that I was wasting his time and so would not allow dad to call again.

At 11.00pm, Dad walked into my bedroom, took one look at me and said, "I am calling the doctor and no arguments".

At 11.30pm, Dr Davidson immediately diagnosed classic gallbladder symptoms and told me that he would be phoning *Mr Grace at the hospital to get me an appointment a.s.a.p. I was then given morphine to take the pain away.

On Monday 24 April at 8am I was met by a horrendous sight when I walked into the bathroom and viewed my reflection in the mirror. The pressure of battling against the pain had caused the blood vessels in the whites of my eyes to haemorrhage and my skin had turned yellow overnight. I looked and felt horrific!

At 8.30am Dr Davidson phoned to tell me that I was to go and see Mr Grace at 2pm. That afternoon I was x-rayed with the results showing that my gallbladder had become gangrenous. Mr Grace also told me he would be writing to my regular GP, telling him in no uncertain terms that he had totally misdiagnosed my symptoms.

On Tuesday 25 April, I underwent an operation to remove my gall bladder and gallstones; over 140 of the little blighters to be exact.

By this time, they could have chopped my head off; all I wanted was to be rid of the constant pain in my abdomen and back.

As I made myself comfortable Olive, the lady in the next bed, asked me what I was in for.

"Gallstones," I said.

"That's what I came in for three weeks ago and I am still waiting for the operation. I have got to have a lumbar puncture this afternoon to find out what the problem is."

Olive's comment absolutely terrified me. The thought of having to have a lumbar puncture filled me with dread, so I went and hid in the toilets trying to compose myself. The next minute the door opened and Sister stood there.

"I've been looking for you everywhere. Whatever's the matter?"

I then told her what had been said to me and that I was absolutely terrified. Sister explained that I would be having a straightforward Cholecystectomy, so I would not need a lumber puncture.

What should have been a six day stay in hospital turned into a three week stay due to complications arising from the surgery and the internal "matter" that was around the site of my operation.

My abiding memory from this stay in hospital was a Staff Nurse who always worked on the night shift. I named her Amazing Grace because this is what she sang all the time and she was most definitely an Earth Angel, God bless her!

I can remember one particular night "shuffling" to the toilet, bent double because of the pain in my back and down my leg. Amazing Grace saw me and said, "Straighten up!"

"I have such a pain in my back and going right down into my leg; it is preventing me from walking properly," I replied.

Obviously alarm bells rang somewhere because the next minute all hell seemed to break loose and I was immediately escorted back to bed.

Amazing Grace was astute enough to realise what was happening and knew that they had to operate immediately because a week had passed since my operation.

What happened next is a blur, because it all happened so quickly. I heard something mentioned about them having to perform an operation immediately where I lay on my bed. I was given a lump of wood to bite on, whilst Amazing Grace held one of my hands and dear Olive, who by this time had been diagnosed with liver cancer, held my other hand.

It was discovered that I had developed abscesses around the gall bladder operation site, which was causing referred pain in my leg.

Although I had been suffering from a severe temperature for several days, the surgeon had told me that it was the internal bruising from the operation that was making me feel so ill.

The moment the doctor opened the end of my surgical scar with a pair of surgical scissors the relief was instant as all the "filth" that had accumulated internally was released

What was meant to be a six day stay in hospital turned into three weeks, because *Sister Hudson would not allow me go to home when there was only my dad to look after me. Even then, I was only allowed home on the proviso that the District nurse visited me every day to change the dressing on my operation site, which had been kept open.

Olive passed away three days after I left hospital. God bless her for she was definitely an Earth Angel.

Once again, during this three week stay in hospital, Chris proved her friendship to me by picking Dad up every day (sometimes twice a day) and bringing him to the hospital to visit me, all without asking.

I was discharged from hospital on 12 May, still feeling quite poorly.

It was not until years later that I realised that had the abscesses burst, I would not be here now. I have always credited Amazing Grace, God Bless her, for saving my life.

May Blossom? Yes, all my "troubles" were over.

The month of May was come when every lusty heart beginneth to blossom and to bring forth fruit

Sir Thomas Mallory
English author 1470-1471

1974 - March

In the Bonded Warehouse where I worked there were two companies; one company bottled and packed spirits and the second company, British Rail, as it was then, handled and shipped the goods.

I had been off work with the flu when my good friend Lou took me down to work to collect my wages. There was no banking system then and your wages were paid to you by hand in a little brown envelope.

As I started to walk across the yard to the office, I noticed Gerald Edward Elson, otherwise known as "Pip", staring at me intently. As I drew level with him, he asked where I had been. I told him that I had been off ill with the flu.

"Oh! I would have sent you some flowers if I had known," he replied.

My response to this remark was to give him (in Pips words) a look as if he was "off his trolley". I just thought it was a very strange remark to make.

The following Monday (11th) I went back to work and everywhere I looked, Pip was there! Little did I know he was trying to pluck up courage to ask me out!

Walking back from a tea break, Pip greeted me with the following words, "What would you say if I asked you out"?

I was quite taken aback, but somehow I seemed to answer, "Yes, ok", and that was it. Pip just turned away and walked off, leaving me there in total bewilderment. "Well what was that all about then?" I thought.

Two days went by and it was as if Pip had disappeared off the face of the Earth. He was nowhere to be seen. Had I imagined it? Had he really asked me out? These were the words that kept going around and around in my head and the realisation that I wanted it to be true was the most surprising thing for me.

On Wednesday 13th March at 8am, as I walked into work, Steve Clark, Pip's best mate, told me that Pip was in the booking office and that he was leaving on Friday. Summoning up all my courage I knocked on the office door, strode in and said, "Are you taking me out then, or were you joking?"

I will never forget the look of sheer terror on Pip's face. A long time after that, he told me that had there been a door the other side of the office, he would have shot through it! He also told me that the real reason he had kept his distance was because he felt he was not "good enough" for me. This statement completely shook me and I could not comprehend why he would think that.

I later discovered that Pip had a huge inferiority complex and believed that everyone else was better than him. How wrong can a man be, or anyone come to that? We are all God's children and in my eyes no better or worse than anyone else.

On Wednesday 27 March, Pip said, "If I asked you to marry me, what would you say?"

I said "Yes" immediately and that was it. I knew that I had met my Soul-mate at long last. I was 27 and Pip was 30.

On Saturday 13 April we got engaged. Pip had asked Dad for my hand in marriage and he was delighted. He loved Pip as a son and always treated him as such.

At the time that we decided to get engaged, "our house" (Dad's and mine) went on the market for £700.00.

Pip, being the wonderful man that he is, decided we should live with my dad after we got married. He felt it was not right to ask me to leave my dad on his own, because we had been through too much together.

He was right; I could no more have left my dad to live on his own than I could have flown single-handedly to the moon.

1975

Saturday 17 May was our wedding day. Even the wet and windy weather could not have dampened my spirits. I was going to be marrying the man that I had been waiting for all of my life - Gerald Edward Elson - and at long last my life was complete, or very nearly.

The only sad part of my wedding day and the pre-wedding preparations was of not having Mum there to help me choose my wedding dress, and everything else that goes into organising one of the most important days of one's life.

At 9.00am, when I was sitting at the hairdressers having my hair done, a voice on the radio suddenly said, "Margaret Wright, are you there? I hope so, because I have a message for you from Pip. He wants you to know he loves you very much and cannot wait to marry you this afternoon!"

I was rendered speechless and could not believe what I had just heard. Pip had just told me and the listening public that he loved me and could not wait to marry me. It was totally alien to Pip's nature, but he had and he did tell everyone that he loved me!

At 2.55pm as I walked into the lounge, Dad took one look at me in my wedding dress and swiftly walked out the door. I stood there feeling slightly hurt as to why he had not commented on how I looked. It was because he couldn't. The sight of me in my wedding dress had filled him with such emotion that he had to go outside away from prying eyes and try to compose himself.

We were both missing Mum and although neither of us spoke of this, we were both aware of her absence.

At 3.00pm coming out of the front door, I was greeted by a crowd of people in the street clapping and cheering. This made me feel so very special and left me with a wonderful memory.

Dad and I got into the waiting wedding car to be promptly asked by the driver, "Are you not carrying any flowers?"

In my haste to get to church, I had forgotten my bouquet of deep Red roses.

We had forty people at the sit down meal in the afternoon and at night another eighty came and helped us celebrate. What a day and night to remember!

We had been buying alcoholic drink for the last twelve months and with Dad's allowance from the brewery a good time was had by all.

Unbeknownst to me at the time, Dad drank a bottle of whisky, which was surprising as he always liked a pint and nothing else.

When it came to saying goodbye, (we were going to Jersey for our honeymoon), Dad and I broke down sobbing in each other's arms, even though I was returning in a week! However, it had been such an emotion packed day that it was inevitable that tears would result and the guests literally had to prise us apart.

A week later we were back and as we turned the corner at the top of the street, there was Dad waiting on the doorstep.

As soon as I stepped out of the taxi, Dad told me how much he had missed me and also how poorly he had been. The morning after our wedding he had looked in the mirror to see that his skin had turned yellow. He had promptly gone to the doctor and been diagnosed with jaundice.

I burst out laughing at this and said, "Do you not think that maybe it was all the whisky that you consumed that caused you to go yellow?"

Dad sheepishly agreed that maybe it was.

1976

On Thursday 1 April, Dad retired from work.

On Tuesday 27 April, our son Grahame was born and Dad duly adored him. He was such a proud grandad and even more so when our daughter Cheryl arrived on his birthday, 12 March 1978. We all felt that this was a special birthday gift from Mum, their first and only granddaughter, but equally, so was Grahame, our first born.

(Derek had become a dad to a son, Darren, in September 1970)

Dad adored all of his grandchildren and they adored him. To say that my dad was the proudest grandad in history is an understatement. His fellow choir members used to tell me that no one had grandchildren like my dad. This made me so happy, but it was also tinged with the regret that Mum had not been able to experience what being a grandma entailed. This was her dearest wish and she was always saying, "For goodness sake, hurry up and make me a grandma," but that wish was never fulfilled.

The intervening years between 1976 and 1991 were spent being a wife, mother and looking after Dad. I also had numerous jobs; cleaner, school dinner lady, cook and shop assistant.

1988

On Thursday 5 May at a routine "top and tail" examination, the doctor said, "There appears to be a lump here in your right breast. I will make you an appointment at the hospital for you to have a mammogram, just to be on the safe side."

To say that I was shocked is not an exaggeration.

On Monday 16 May whilst sitting in the waiting room at the hospital, *Mrs Markfield who, like me, was also called Margaret, told me that she too was there to have a lump investigated in her breast. How very uncanny; two Margarets and both with breast lumps!

I was then called in to see the consultant, only to find it was a junior doctor (who barely looked out of nappies) who was going to be examining me. Oh well, "Lie back and think of England" was my immediate thought.

After what seemed an age of me "posing" and him prodding, he said, "I will go and tell Mr Grace what I have found."

Seeing the look of shock on my face, he quickly retracted and said, "I mean, what I haven't found" and quickly exited the room.

I sat on the side of the bed with my head full of thoughts of radical mastectomies, death and dying, Pip losing me, the children losing their mum and Dad losing his daughter, just like Mum, to breast cancer.

I was simply devastated and wanted to break down and cry, but Pip was waiting outside for me so I had to maintain my composure for fear of worrying him.

Mr Grace walked into the room and promptly told me that they were going to "Err on the side of caution". I was to go back in the following October to have another mammogram and see if anything had developed. Mr Grace quickly reassured me by saying, "As yet, they have not found anything sinister".

Three months on and I felt like the Sword of Damocles was being held over my head. I was becoming paranoid about cancer developing and every morning and every night I would be prodding and poking to see what I could "find".

One particular night, I had gone to bed early and as I lay reading I lifted my arm over my head and subconsciously started to "feel" my armpit; this is where Mum's cancer had started as a little pea shaped lump).

"Oh my God," I thought. There was quite a firm lump. I started shaking and crying, absolutely petrified that all my worries had now manifested into the real thing. I convinced myself I was going to die.

Pip held me in his arms trying to calm me down, but his constant words of "You're fine; you're not going anywhere," went totally unnoticed!

I was beside myself with anxiety and could not think of anything other than my mortality. My nightmare had become a reality!

As Pip sat holding me, I felt a sudden "presence" fill the room. Standing in front of me was Mum and she had come to give me a message.

"You are fine and have nothing to worry about. Don't you remember me telling you that I hoped I had done all the suffering for you too?"

I did remember and suddenly I was standing under a waterfall and as the water flowed down my body, all my fears and doubts were washed away.

I was going to be alright. I was not going to die and mum had just told me so.

The next day I made an appointment to see the doctor and he was to tell me that it was a "fatty" lump that was nothing to worry about.

I gave humble thanks to the "great man" himself that day, but I still had to go back in October for another mammogram.

On Monday 10 October I went for my second mammogram and had to go back the following week for the results.

On Monday 17 October, Mr Grace's registrar informed me that they had not "found" anything, hinted that it had all been a waste of time and promptly walked out of the room. I sat there stunned and Pip, who had been allowed to come in with me said, "Well, that was a waste of time".

I sat there in stunned silence, too shocked to speak. Had that really happened? Had he really dismissed me in that way? It was at this point that I started to get angry. How dare he? Did he not realise what I had been through these last five months of uncertainty?

I was so upset that I began to cry. Pip could not understand why I was crying when I had just been given the all clear. To my mind this was a man thing, having no idea what it meant to be told that you did not have breast cancer and for this man to be so dismissive, was more than I could take at that time.

A few weeks later I was reading a column in a magazine and the female writer was telling of her experience of having a mammogram and being told, like me, that it had been a waste of time.

*Mary had written: "Any of you women out there who have suffered the same fate as me, stand up and be counted; do not let these doctors get away with it".

With her comments in mind, I went back to see the doctor and told her of my disgust at the way I had been treated and that my intention was to make sure that this whole sorry scenario would not happen to another woman.

*Dr Elliot said that she would write to Mr Grace on my behalf, stating what I had told her. The following week I was called back to the surgery and shown a letter of apology, ensuring they would make sure that this kind of incident never happened again. I know that today there is a more sympathetic approach to what is every woman's nightmare, so hopefully we did some good.

*Mrs Markfield? Unfortunately Margaret died and that was not only very sad, but also very scary and, beggars the question; why her and not me? No answer, but these words immediately sprung to mind;

"There but for the grace of God go I"

You pray in your distress and in your need, would that you might pray also in the fullness of your joy and in your days of abundance

- Kahlil Gibran -

1991

In February I started work as a domestic at a local boarding school. It was whilst working there that I had my first real spiritual "experience".

Each domestic was responsible for looking after their own unit and I was working away in mine when I heard a voice say, "*Jayne's daughter has taken an overdose".

I spun round to see who had spoken in my ear, but there was no one there!

"Jayne's daughter has taken an overdose and you have to go and tell her!"

I stood rooted to the spot, shocked and in total disbelief at what I "thought" I had just heard. I could not comprehend how I had heard this voice when there was no one else visible in the room, much the same as when mum had "spoken" to me!!

"You have to go and tell Jayne her daughter's life is in danger."

There it was again, only this time I "knew" that it was a message from beyond!

I have no recollection as to how I conveyed this message to Jayne, but what I can remember is Jayne trying to contact her daughter by phone. Getting no reply she immediately went home to find that her daughter had taken enough tablets for it to be a borderline situation between life and death.

I still wonder to this day why I was given this message. I barely knew Jayne, or her family. Someone "up there" did not want this girl to die and used me to save her life and for that I will be eternally grateful.

If the only prayer you ever say in your entire life is "Thank You", it will be enough

*- Meister Eckhart (1260-1328)
German Dominican Mystic -*

My second "experience" happened again whilst I was still at this school.

On 1 April, Pip was working nights at British Rail and I had gone to bed about 11.00pm. I must have been in some kind of dream state because the next minute I saw, what can only be described as, a "fluffy white cloud" floating up the bedroom wall. I shot up in bed and "knew" instantly that someone had died.

Had Pip had an accident? What about Dad? No, I heard him cough.

It was then I was "told" to look at the clock. It was 11.20pm.

I stood at the bedroom window waiting for the phone to ring to give me bad news. By midnight there had been no phone call and no knocks at the door. It was at this point that I decided that I must have imagined it all, that it was probably a dream, so I got back into bed and promptly fell asleep.

At 6am on Tuesday 2 April, Pip came home from working nights, had his breakfast and went straight to bed. At that time, I did not recall the event from the night before.

At 8.20am the Deputy Head came into my unit and told me that my dad was on the phone, wishing to speak to me. My immediate thought was that Grahame or Cheryl was poorly, but Dad had rung to tell me that "Father-in-law" had passed away. By this I thought he meant Derek's father-in-law, but it was Pip's dad. Dad asked me whether I could inform Betty, Pip's sister, who also worked as a domestic at the school.

Pip's Dad, for whatever reason, had taken it into his head many years before that Pip (Gerald) was not his own birth child and had banned him from going to his house, which is why I was so surprised by the news.

I went and relayed the message to Betty, but as I was walking back to my unit, Dad's words suddenly registered: "Pip's Dad has died".

This stopped me dead in my tracks. Was this the connection to what happened the previous night; the premonition that someone had died at 11.20pm?

I went back to Betty and asked her to ring her sister to enquire at what time their Dad had died. It was 11.20pm!

Why should I see this man's soul going over? We had not seen him in ten years so why should I have witnessed his passing?

It turned out that the last thing that this man ever said was "Gerald". He was calling out for his only son as he departed this world for the next, so why did he not call for him in this life, not as he was leaving it?

1992 - June

Dad had been poorly for a good few years with smoking related illnesses. He had started smoking when he was 12 and he was now 81, so he had had 39 years of cigarettes and the last 30 years of smoking a pipe.

I can remember the winter of 1982, which was quite severe. We had had central heating installed in the summer of 1981 and this proved to be a Godsend, with Dad having to spend six weeks in bed suffering from bronchial pneumonia. Even so, he would sit in bed with his unlit pipe in his mouth, waiting until he could get to light it again.

These illnesses had gradually become so intense that in late 1990, due to oedema in his legs and body, he could not stand for any length of time. Having to take water tablets meant that he could not venture far and so was not able to attend choir practice. This was especially hard on him as he loved his choir; it was one of his reasons for living.

I suggested that maybe he could go to choir practice and sit down, but his reply was very terse.

Cheryl, his little nurse, used to bathe his ulcerated legs until in the end it became too much and we had to have the District Nurse come in and do it for us. Dad hated this. He said it robbed him of his dignity.

On Tuesday 2 June 1992 at 2pm, Dad suddenly said, "I think I will get into bed for a while" and then promptly said that he needed to go to the toilet. I went out of the room so that he could use his commode. Half an hour later when I went back in he said "Still haven't been" and he never did.

I instinctively knew that this was the start of the end. He was accepting the inevitable; his death. His whole demeanour had changed over the previous weeks. He had basically lost interest in everything, he had lost his appetite and he seemed to be sleeping more.

One of the hardest things I have ever had to do was tell Grahame and Cheryl their treasured Grandad was extremely poorly and would not be with us for much longer.

It also transpired that a couple of days before, Dad had got Cheryl to sort out his belongings and decide who was having what.

Cheryl had done this without an inkling of what was going to happen to "her" grandad.

Dad was the original male chauvinist; the women were there to "do" and the man went out to work!

On the night bridging 2-3 June, I had requested that I be on my own with Dad as I knew that it would be the last time that I would be able to look after him in this life.

Around 3.00am, he suddenly opened his eyes, looked past me (and the strange thing was I knew that Mum was standing there by my side) and said, "I have had enough Mother. I cannot take anymore. I am coming home!"

Pip got up at 5.00am and came and sat with me, to be followed by Grahame and Cheryl at 6.00am.

Dad passed over peacefully at precisely 8.15am. He just allowed death to enfold him and quietly slipped away with Grahame, Cheryl and myself at his bedside. Pip was too upset to be there and could not bear to watch this man, who had been more of a father to him than his own Dad, slip away.

When the doctor confirmed that Dad had "gone", he turned to us all as a family and said that it had been a privilege to be a part of what, to him, was an old fashioned death. By this he meant that all the family were there to be with their beloved as they departed this world for the next.

The doctor then turned to me and said, "I hope that your death will be as peaceful and accepting as your father's has been."

I thanked him, but told him that I was not planning on going anywhere as yet!

At 9.00am on Monday 8 June, we were at High Bank Road Chapel again, only this time it was for Dad's funeral.

We had never discussed what kind of funeral he wanted, so as a family we decided that we would like it to be a celebration of his life. One of the hymns that I chose was "Amazing Grace" and his fellow choir members were there in full voice and paid Harold a huge compliment in the way that they sang for him.

As we started to leave the chapel, they started to sing a tribute hymn, Tydi-a-Roddiast. This is a piece especially written for top tenors and at the end there are four Amens, which build until the very last Amen, which is full pitch. I asked that we stop and listen to this note and as it reached its crescendo I could see Dad laughing and heard him say, "By gad they sang that well", which made me smile.

The committal commenced at 10.30am at Bretby Crematorium, which did not exist when Mum died in 1969.

I had chosen a recording of the choir singing Morti Christie. This is one of my favourite hymns and Dad's voice could be heard ringing out as the curtains enclosed his coffin in a fitting tribute to the man and his music.

Peter and Tommy, two of the choir members, came to the crematorium for Dad's committal. Peter was a dear friend and had faithfully picked Dad up twice a week for as long as I can remember and taken him to choir practice. Tommy had stood next but one to Dad in the choir for over forty years and was also a close friend.

After the committal service, Peter and Tommy told us how Dad used to reminisce about his beloved grandchildren; how Grahame always sat with him to watch TV and programmes like Quincy, Murder She Wrote and Columbo and how Cheryl, his little nurse, tended to his every need!

Tommy was to tell me that Dad had phoned him the week before and told him that he was "ready to go", that he'd "had enough". This was quite a shock, but somehow it explained his remark to me on the Monday night prior to his death on the Wednesday.

Last thing at night I always used to go into his room and say, "Night, night. See you in the morning" and ruffle his hair. His reply "You might do!" stopped me dead in my tracks, but I felt too frightened to ask him what he meant.

After Dad's funeral the undertakers asked us whether we wanted to take his ashes to be scattered at Markeaton Crematorium in Derby alongside Mum. It was the one thing that I could not do for him. It was too final. The thought of carrying my Dad in a box filled me with dread and Cheryl and Grahame felt the same, so we asked the undertakers to do it for us.

People would stop me in the street afterwards and tell me how much they had enjoyed Dad's funeral, how it had been so uplifting and how well his Choir had sung for him. These sentiments made me feel so proud that we had looked after him in death with as much care as we had in life.

On Saturday 21 November, the Gresley Male Voice Choir Celebrity Concert took place at Burton Town Hall. On this night, the men of the choir paid homage to Harold in a way that would have made my dad so very proud.

Dad was a stickler for things being done in the right way and his beloved choir was no different, especially at choir practice. He was not averse to speaking his mind if he thought anyone was not paying attention to Roy (the conductor) and he would tell them, in no uncertain terms, what he thought of their behaviour. Roy made this comment on the night and said how much he missed Harold for his unending strength and support, not only for himself but for the choir also.

In the interval I was invited onto the stage to accept a Long Service Award on behalf of Dad and as I got up from my seat to walk to the stage, the men of the choir rose as one in acknowledgment to Harold. This unexpected show of respect was my undoing. Struggling in vain with my emotions, I accepted a Lifetime Member Award in recognition of Dad's commitment to the choir over the previous thirty seven years.

As a final tribute they sang his funeral hymn Tydi-a-Roddiast. Thank you Gresley Male Voice Choir for the wonderful tribute paid to the memory of Harold, my dad!

And so another part of my life was over, but Dad would still play a big part in the next.

Dad, your guiding hand on my shoulder will remain with me forever

- Author Unknown -

Part Two

My Spiritual Awakening

To
Reiki Master/Teacher
&
"Mags Wise Owl"
Spiritual Teacher
&
Beyond!

A Testament to our Spiritual Friendship

By Paul Thomas

Firstly, whilst on my spiritual journey, I've encountered many who have tried aimlessly to lead me away from my path. It is difficult looking for something and not knowing what you are looking for. Some call it soul searching.

Part of my journey took me to a little Spiritualist church in Burton-on-Trent, where after many failed attempts to visit, I finally plucked up the courage, along with a bit of scepticism. I was greeted with a very warm welcome by two lovely people, Margaret and Cheryl. Unknown to me, they were mother and daughter.

After several visits, I very much looked forward to going. However, that soon changed when Margaret and Cheryl were no longer there. My intuition told me that it was not for me anymore. So I left, only to wonder why they'd gone and hoped that one day I could meet them again.

I guess the Divine Source was listening to me. One day in Burton shopping centre I caught a glimpse of them, but I wasn't sure, so I shouted and to my delight it was mum and daughter! It was then that I realised it wasn't the church I missed; it was Margaret and Cheryl.

From then on our spiritual connection grew stronger. Little did I know then how big a part Margaret would play in my life and I in hers.

Now, despite being many miles away, spiritually I stand beside you always. When you need me, you only have to think of me and I call, as you already know. So, as my testament to you, I thank God for putting you into my life, for sharing your love, light and many life experiences with me.

You are truly an Earth Angel and my spiritual soul mate.

I give to you many blessings from my heart.

Paul xx

"Each friend represents a world in us, a world possibly not born until they arrive, and it is only by this meeting that a new world is born."

- Anais Nin -

"He's Here You Know!"

These are Pip words when he smelled Dad's tobacco in the hall, prompting him to walk into the lounge and say, "He's here you know".

"Who?" I asked.

"Your Dad," replied Pip. "Can't you smell his tobacco?"

I could not and never have. Dad shows himself to me in other ways; ruffling my hair, brushing my cheek with a kiss and always with the feeling of "knowing" that he is still around.

The love that we had for each other could not be broken by his death. It was far too strong and goes beyond the veil to other dimensions, past lives and other planets. The connection is there and always will be no matter where we reside in the Universe.

Love you dad forever!

There's something like a line of gold thread running through a man's words when he talks to his daughter, and gradually over the years it gets to be long enough for you to pick up in your hands and weave into a cloth that feels like love itself

- John Gregory Brown -
Decorations in a Ruined Cemetery, 1994

2002- 2009:
My Journey to the Present Day

2002

At 6.00am on Thursday 5 September, the phone rang. My subconscious was telling me to wake up and answer it.

It was Chris ringing me to tell me that her mum had died in the night after suffering an aneurism. I could not absorb the information, because it was just not possible. At 87-years-old, this wonderful lady who loved to laugh and joke had died when she had not even been poorly.

Mrs Tatton, a true Earth Angel, had been like a second mum to me and now she too had died. I was devastated, not only for Chris but for myself. The thought of not seeing this wonderful lady again was unimaginable.

2003 - January

Struggling to come to terms with the grief of losing her mum, I tentatively suggested to Chris that maybe we could go to a Spiritualist church, just to see. After all, it was her mum who had first taken me and that was the turning point in helping me to cope with my loss.

At 6.00pm on Sunday 12 January, we were at the Spiritualist Church in Derby. We sang hymns, said a few prayers and then the medium stood up and said, "I have a gentleman here. Oh, no I don't! I have a lady who has just pushed her way to the front. 'I'm Doris and I want you to give a message to my daughter'".

The medium then looked straight at Chris and said, "Your mum's here".

From that day Chris never looked back, receiving such a profound message from her mum was just what Chris needed. Her mum was still around and watching over her. It was also at this point in time that I was first given proof that "they" do listen to what we say and what we talk about.

On three consecutive Sundays in a row, different mediums stood on the platform and repeated word for word our conversations as we journeyed to the church. On the third Sunday we decided to lay a "trap", but we lost!!!! We engaged in a complicated conversation about what was happening in my life at that time. We included some really obscure quotes and I can remember us laughing and saying they would not be able to repeat this, but they did!!!

It was beyond rhyme or reason how someone could literally repeat word for word what we had discussed on our journey to the church three Sundays in a row. There was only one explanation; Angels!

Over the next few months we carried on attending church, but the only message was for me: "You are a Healer".

2004

On Sunday 4 January, I decided that I would attend a Spiritualist church that was local to me. The very first Sunday, the resident medium described my dad to me and said that "he" had followed me through the door and was standing behind me.

In April, I started to "sit" in circle for the very first time in my life and within a matter of weeks I was to meet my Spirit Guide, Saskatchewan.

I was deep into meditation when I felt myself going through a waterfall. As I emerged through the other side I could see a Red Indian standing there, almost as if he was waiting for me. He then beckoned me to follow him. We started running through the woods (at this point I knew that we were in Canada) eventually coming out into a clearing and before me stood an Indian camp.

Two Feathers (he told me that was his name as we were running through the forest) took me through the camp to where a Medicine Man was seated outside of his Tepee. "He" then stood up and took me on a tour of his camp and, stopping and pointing at a fast flowing river, he said, "Saskatchewan" and then pointed at his chest. I knew instantly that he was telling me that was his name. I then told him mine, but he already knew!

I could not wait to get home and see what Saskatchewan meant. I knew that it was a place in Canada, but something was telling me that it translated to something else. I was speechless. Saskatchewan: meaning; Rapid River (Indian translation).

I was beside myself with excitement and could not wait to go back and sit in circle in the hope of "meeting" Saskatchewan again. I was not disappointed!

A couple of weeks later, walking around a local market, I heard a voice say, "I am here" and, turning around, there he was exactly as I had seen him in meditation. Even more spookily, who was standing next to him? Two Feathers, of course!

Over the following weeks my connection with Saskatchewan became stronger and he started showing me where some of the people sitting in circle had various problems, manifesting into the physical body.

After we were called back from meditation, we sat and discussed what we had seen, heard or experienced. When it came to my turn I was very reluctant to say what I had been told. After all, who would believe me?

Imagine my shock and surprise when I related to *Peter what I had been shown, as in a block of negativity in his Sacral and Solar Plexus region. He confirmed that he had been suffering with diverticulitis, a debilitating condition for many years and that he had also been diagnosed with diabetes the previous week.

It was to get even better. The following week I was shown a metal rod going up *Ruth's spine. Ruth confirmed that she had had this metal rod in her back for numerous years owing to a degenerative spinal condition.

I was totally overawed by what was happening to me, but over the next few weeks the strength of our connection was to increase.

In August of the same year, I was at a local bowls' match when, looking over at one of the bowlers, I could see a "dark spot" around his kidney area. I had to blink and look again, not really believing what I was being shown, but a dark area surrounding his kidneys was visible to my psychic eye.

Just then, his wife Edna came over to where I was sitting and started to tell me that Gary had not been feeling well for the last few weeks and he was due to go and have a scan the following Wednesday to find out why. I was deeply puzzled as to why Edna had given me this information as I had barely spoken to either of them beforehand.

Edna rang me the following week to tell me that Gary had been diagnosed with kidney cancer. Gary passed away in the October leaving his wife Edna desolate and his family inconsolable.

In October, I had my first encounter with the "dark side" whilst sitting in the Circle. Unbeknownst to the rest of us, we had a person sitting in circle that was connecting with the dark side!

Going into meditation, I had felt dad's presence very close beside me. I did not question it. I felt him ruffle my hair and kiss my cheek. The next second I saw - what I can only describe as - "black things" coming towards me at great speed and then literally knocking me straight back in my chair. To say that I was deeply disturbed by this "encounter" is an understatement. I was trembling and very upset and, even more disturbingly, I knew where they had come from.

At this time in my life I had no conception of grounding and protection, leaving myself open to all and sundry "coming" in and attacking my aura.

(An explanation to auras, energy field, grounding and protecting will be given in part three)

> ***The aura given out by a person or object is as much a part of them as their flesh***
>
> *~ Lucian Freud ~*

In late November, Cheryl and I went to visit Edna to see how she was coping with life without Gary. As we sat talking, I was aware of Gary walking by the lounge door. I looked straight at Cheryl and I knew from her face that she had seen him too. Edna saw the look and immediately asked what the matter was. I was reluctant to say at first for fear of upsetting her, but then I heard Gary's voice say, "Tell her".

As I told Edna what we had seen (a shadow passing the door), her face was incredulous. Edna had also been "seeing" this shadow, but had thought that it was her imagination.

In November, the Annual General Meeting was held at the church and I reluctantly took the "Chair". I did this to ensure that the church remained open for those who needed it. This was a decision that unfortunately was to cost me dearly health wise.

From the moment that I took the chair it was a constant battle with people wanting to have their say without wanting the responsibility.

Totally oblivious to the importance of grounding and protecting, visitors to the church would constantly drain me of all my energy. There were also other ongoing issues and battles between people within the church, which proved to be very stressful.

Eventually, chronic fatigue and, as mentioned a little further on, an abscess beneath my wisdom tooth caused me to leave the church.

On Friday 24 December, we held a Candlelit Carol Service at the church. The medium started to give her message from the rostrum.

"Margaret, your mum is here and she is asking me to remind you of the Christmases you spent together cooking and baking in the kitchen. She wants you to know she will be there with you in spirit tomorrow, looking on and 'helping'."

I mentally asked Mum for a sign to be given to me with 100% proof that she would be there, helping!

At 11.00am on Saturday 25 December, Pip got up from his chair and for the umpteenth time looked out of the front window. His next words took both Cheryl and I by surprise.

"Is that a twenty pound note?"

That was as far as he got. Cheryl was out of the door like a flash and underneath one of the bushes in the front garden was a twenty pound note, folded in half!

The three of us stood looking at each other, not quite believing what Cheryl was holding in her hand; a twenty pound note, lying in the garden, folded in half and looking as if it had been placed there.

There was only one explanation. Mum had heard and answered my prayer. She was still around and watching over us, along with Dad of course!

2005 - March

I started to learn about "spiritual healing" at the church, but after a couple of months I knew that it was not right for me. It was also about this time I started to have problems with a wisdom tooth that was giving me a lot of pain and discomfort. This tooth and *Emily Booth turned out to be another catalyst that helped me on my pathway to Reiki.

Emily had been a Medium in the church for many years, but had sadly passed away just before Christmas

2004. Whilst still at the church, I gave Emily "hands on healing". Her words to me afterwards, "You do not realise how strong you are", went straight over the top of my head. I hadn't got a clue as to what she meant.

On Wednesday 16 March, when I was sitting in the circle, I was asked to sit on the rostrum and "give" messages to the other "sitters". This was all to do with our spiritual development and to help us to connect to "spirit".

As I was sitting on the rostrum, a brilliant white light (like a giant sun) began to shine into my face, causing me to put my hands up to shield my eyes. We were all sitting in candlelight, but when I asked if anyone else could see this light, it was met with a negative. How very strange. I could not comprehend why no one else could see this brilliant white light when it was literally blinding me!

One morning towards the end of April, Pip asked, "Did you see that woman come through the window last night?"

"No," I replied, "Who was it?"

"I don't know. All I know is that she woke me up and then looked at you and promptly went back out of the window."

When Pip related this to Cheryl, she immediately said, "Oh, that was Emily Booth and she has come to get Mum out of the church!"

Emily did get me out of the church, at the beginning of May 2005 to be precise. My wisdom tooth had become infected and I was on antibiotics, but somehow the poison had got into my system, making me really ill. So that was it; Emily had succeeded. I handed in my resignation to the church and immediately felt as if a weight had been lifted off my shoulders.

On Friday 17 June, Chris came for dinner, but unfortunately because she was in so much pain from the recent surgery she had had on her jaw, she was unable to eat, because it was far too painful.

Some little voice inside of me told me to put my hands around her face. Immediately we could both feel the intense "energy" coming through the palms of my hands. Within minutes Chris had gone to "sleep" and when she woke up, the pain had gone. She told me that she thought that I was going to "burn" her face as my hands had been so hot on her skin.

We were both mystified by this inexplicable phenomenon that had occurred, but explanations were to come later the more I advanced on my "Reiki" pathway.

On Thursday 23 June, Pip, Cheryl and I flew out to Majorca and whilst there a "miracle" took place, once more concerning Cheryl.

Cheryl had been diagnosed as having suspected Endometriosis in March of that year and was due back in the September to see the Consultant for further treatment. We had only been in Majorca for two days when Cheryl suddenly had a severe attack of crippling pain, which confined her to bed.

I was guided to do a "healing" on her and was concentrating on this when Cheryl was suddenly aware that Rapid River was standing "watching" over what was happening. He was standing in the hotel balcony doorway overseeing the healing and guiding me subconsciously to where I had to lay my hands on Cheryl.

The next morning Cheryl greeted me with the words, "What the hell have you done to me? I feel worse now than before" and spent the next two days in bed really poorly. I was extremely worried and felt terribly guilty seeing her like this without the knowledge to understand what had happened. I had no concept of what I now know to be a "Healing Crisis" and was totally naive in the knowledge that this was her body's way of rectifying itself and getting rid of all the toxins that were poisoning her and making her so unwell.

The following day Cheryl was completely pain free, which left both of us totally mystified and, once again Cheryl told me that I had got "something special" in my hands.

On Thursday 25 July, I went to have my Aura-Soma read, although beforehand I had no idea what this meant.

As I shook hands with *Grace, she told me that she could see the aura of a healer around me and promptly asked if I was Reiki. I looked at her blankly and said, "No, what is Reiki?"

Grace then explained to me what Reiki was and that when Jesus walked the Earth plane, I had walked with him as one of his healers. I was completely taken aback by her comments and for once in my life was left speechless. How on earth could I, Margaret Ann Elson, have worked with Jesus? That was taking things too far and at that moment in time was totally unbelievable to me! Grace advised me that I needed to look for a Reiki Master a.s.a.p.

Chris Ward, Reiki Master, was the name that jumped out at me as I looked in the phone book. I immediately contacted her and we arranged to meet the following Thursday, 1st August.

Chris met me with a big hug and a lovely smile and I connected straight away with this likeminded soul. Saskatchewan had chosen well.

I started to tell Chris a little bit about myself and when I mentioned Saskatchewan, she looked surprised. The day before, she had looked out into her garden to see a Red Indian standing there looking back at her! She knew he was obviously there for a reason.

Chris had then gone out into the garden and as she walked back noticed a feather hanging in the finest gossamer web just above the conservatory door. She thought it was strange, but decided to take a picture as she knew there was a message there, as yet unexplained.

Rapid River had shown himself and his approval of Chris by leaving his calling card; a feather in a gossamer spider's web attached to the conservatory door.

A month later on Thursday 8 September, I returned to do my Second Degree Reiki.

During the day, Rapid River told me that I would be back for my Reiki Master the following April and he even gave me the date; the 7th, Pip's 63rd birthday.

On Monday 12 September, Cheryl went back to see the Consultant Gynaecologist at the hospital and was given the all clear. This news proved, beyond a shadow of a doubt, that a miracle had taken place in Majorca and it was all down to Rapid River and his Divine Healing presence.

So, once again, Cheryl was playing an important part in helping me to achieve my destiny.

*A mother's love for her child is like
nothing else in the world.*

It knows no law, no pity.

*It dares all things and crushes down
remorselessly all that stands in its path.*

- Agatha Christie -

On Thursday 15 September, my first Reiki client visited. *Lisa was a friend of Edna's son and he had recommended me. A multitude of thoughts whirred around in my head. What if I did it wrong? What if I made a mess of it? I so desperately wanted to do a "healing", but now that it was about to materialise, I felt extremely nervous.

Lisa informed me that she had lost her dad the previous May, 2004 and was still struggling to come to terms with her grief and felt totally lost and alone. Her husband and family were very supportive, but she just wanted to know that her dad was "alright".

As I laid my hands upon Lisa, it was as if I had "been born" to do it. The "Reiki" flowing through my hands felt so natural, with a beautiful loving energy enfolding it. As I stood basking in the throes of this wonderful experience, I suddenly became aware of a "man" standing by my right side. He introduced himself, telling me he was Lisa's dad and that he had come to give her a personal message, with the intention it would be of great comfort to her. He said he was aware of how unhappy she had been since losing him and wanted her to know that he was still around and his message would acknowledge that.

After the healing, I gave Lisa the message from her dad and the change in her was unbelievable; tears of joy tinged with sadness.

I was on such a high after what had happened with Lisa that I wanted to "do" another one straight away, but it was to be the following April before my next one. I was quite frustrated by this, as I wanted to be healing every day!

I had this ludicrous idea that I could do at least five treatments a day, every day and this would allow me to finish work. How stupid and naive was I? There are many lessons that you have to learn in Reiki and this was one of them; patience.

2006

On Friday 7 April, my dream became a reality. I was going to be attuned to Reiki Master Divine Source energy and I was beside myself with excitement!

As Chris started to put the symbols into my upper chakras, the strangest thing happened. I was nailed on the cross and looking down on all these people jeering and throwing stones at me. I felt no pain; all I could hear was my voice saying, "Forgive them Father, for they know not what they do!"

I was then made aware of a huge pair of wings wrapping around me and enfolding me with so much love and compassion that I gave forth a huge sob. Immediately, I was back in the room with Chris beside me and tears were in her eyes. She had witnessed it all. I had not imagined it. It had happened and I was overcome with such powerful emotions that I cried as if my heart was broken.

I had never spoken those words in my life before, so why that day, of all days? I felt then, and still do to this day, that this was Jesus' way of showing me how powerful Divine Source Reiki can be when used for the right reasons.

Christine Ward? Light Worker/Earth Angel in every sense and meaning of the words!

Religion is a set of social and political institutions.

***Spirituality is a private pursuit which may
or may not take place in a church setting***

- D. Patrick Miller -

On Tuesday 25 April, I was regressed to a past life; Egypt, 680 BC. I had a long held fascination with anything and everything to do with Egypt.

My name was Barabbas and I was a slave. I came "through the door" to be met with the sight of Egyptian soldiers and they had come into my village and taken me to work as a slave. The degradation and inhumane treatment that I suffered at the hands of my own people was a lesson that I was to learn again in this life, only on a much smaller scale.

We were kept in appalling conditions in a stinking rat infested hovel, which seemed to invade all of my senses, the dregs of humanity surrounding me with pitiful wailing noises night after night.

I could feel the heat of the searing sun, day after day, as we were forced to work in harsh conditions in the middle of the desert. Constantly whipped and beaten, I could feel every lash as it sliced across my back.

I was then moved forward in time and I could see myself inside a Royal Palace, once more as a slave. I had no family to speak of. My sister Miriam, I had not seen in years, ever since the soldiers came and took me away. I had no recollection of my parents whatsoever.

I was taken forward to my deathbed. Oh what bliss. I could actually feel the relief that, at long last, I was going to escape from this pitiless life of servitude. I was going to escape and the only way to do that was to die!

As I lay there waiting for death to enfold me, I became aware of a beautiful "white light" shining and shimmering in front of me, almost as if it was reaching out for me. Then, I was in purgatory, confronted by the most hideous of faces; vile, evil faces that were screaming profanities at me.

How on earth had I got there? More to the point, how was I going to get out? I could feel panic welling up into my heart and lungs, suffocating me and preventing me from breathing. And then I heard a voice telling me to turn and go to the light! Dad's voice; yes, it was Dad's voice and he was telling me to "turn and go to the light".

A shaft of the most pure and Divine White Light was coming down before me and I gleefully ran towards it.

My next recollection was of going up in an anti-clockwise[1] direction. Up and up and then, I was through and before me on lily pads were thousands upon thousands of babies waiting to be reincarnated into their next life; And who was standing there waiting for me? Why, Dad of course! My dad was there with arms outstretched, smiling and waiting to greet me.

At that point Tony brought me "back" and told me that I had scared the life out of him when he realised that I was in purgatory.

On Thursday 27 April, my second client *Sally visited me.

In meditation beforehand, Rapid River had shown me three areas of concern; her brow, sacral and base chakras. Using the pendulum, I was given confirmation that these chakras were all blocked with negativity.

Discussing what had occurred during the healing, Sally informed me that she was under the care of the hospital with an ongoing eye problem and was due back at the hospital the following week for a check up. I asked Sally if she was having problems with her periods, but her reply was, "Not really, just heavier than usual" I suggested that maybe she should pay her GP a visit just to check everything was ok.

---

[1] Anti clockwise; Going "up" in an anti-clockwise rotation leaves all negativity endured in that lifetime behind, enabling you to learn new lessons in your next reincarnation.

I was also given a message for Sally. She would be promoted at work, move house (which I described) and I was "shown" her holding a young toddler.

On Friday 28 April, I received an email from Sally to say that she had been back to the hospital and they were very pleased with the improvement in her eyes and were even talking of discharging her if the improvement continued.

Sally did visit her doctor as advised and after having various tests and a scan, a tumour was diagnosed in her cervix. She had to undergo a prolonged course of chemotherapy, which meant that she would not be able to have children naturally. This fact alone was terribly upsetting for her and her husband.

The prognosis was not good, but I never doubted. I absolutely refused to believe that Sally was going to die and throughout this arduous battle she was constantly in my thoughts and prayers.

Saturday 20 May was my first Reiki healing with what I knew to be a cancer related illness. In deep meditation before Doreen arrived, Rapid River showed me a dark area surrounding her sacral/base chakra. He also showed himself dressed from head to toe in buckskin and wearing a full Indian feathered headdress. I was puzzled by this as he had always shown himself wearing a "Buffalo" headdress with a beaded vest and leather trousers. I was soon to discover when he dressed in this way he meant "business"!

Doreen arrived at 11am and was incredibly anxious. She felt as though she had been given a death sentence after being told that her secondary cancer was "too big" to operate on.

As we sat talking, I was shown the cancer close to her ovary on her right hand side. When I asked Doreen to verify this, her answer was a puzzled "Yes".

Within minutes of starting to channel the energy, I was made aware that Doreen had gone to "sleep" and her emotions started to be released. Laying my hands over the site of the tumour, the energy coming through my hands changed and became icy cold.

I was also given a message that she was to surround herself with yellow, as this was the colour that would help her to heal.

Doreen was to go on her "Sacred Reiki Journey" witnessing beautiful shining lights and experiencing a deep burning sensation in her leg. It was over an hour later before I was allowed to call her back to reality.

The healing was to prove very powerful, very intense and the change in Doreen after the healing was in marked contrast to how she had been when she arrived. She felt totally calm and at peace.

I am the Lord that healeth thee

- Exo. 15:26b -

On Saturday 17 June, Doreen brought her mum Gwen to see me and once again Rapid River showed himself in his full ceremonial regalia.

Two days previously, Gwen had been diagnosed with advanced lung cancer and told she had only a matter of weeks to live. She was absolutely terrified and quite literally did not know what to expect.

What a beautiful gentle soul she was and I reassured her that she had nothing to fear. As I laid my hands on her, two things happened in quick succession; Gwen went on her Sacred Reiki Journey and a man who was in spirit came and stood by my side showing me a picture of Gwen and him riding bikes. He said that he was Gwen's husband Jock and this picture was from when they were courting and to please tell Gwen this when she woke up. He also asked me to tell Gwen that she was "not to have it" and that when the time came he would be there waiting for her. She had nothing to fear.

As I sat waiting to "wake" Gwen, she suddenly opened her eyes and said, "I'm back" with the biggest smile on her face and told me that she felt "different" in that she was now calm and felt totally relaxed.

I repeated to Gwen what her husband had told me and she was absolutely delighted with this message and recalled how they used to bike everywhere together. Jock also asked me to remind her about the yellow cardigan. Gwen laughed out loud and told me this was the cardigan she had always worn when they went out biking together. I also repeated the message that she was "not to have it", which turned out to be a huge zap of chemotherapy to try and prolong her life. Gwen had already made her mind up in that she was not going to have it anyway!

On Monday 19 June, Doreen returned to the hospital today to be told the tumour had shrunk so they would be able to operate after all. Doreen and Graham booked a holiday to Jamaica in celebration of this miracle that had occurred.

On Friday 23 June, Doreen rang to tell me that she was taking Gwen for a week's holiday at the seaside so that they could spend precious time together as a family. I was overjoyed at this news and felt privileged to be a part of this joyous occasion.

On Saturday 24 June, as Pip was walking around town, he bumped into an old neighbour of ours and she was to tell him that she had been battling breast cancer the last few months and things were not looking too promising. Pip told her about me and suggested that she came and had Reiki.

*Polly came the following week and as we sat talking about Reiki and how it worked, Rapid River came and stood at her side dressed in his buckskin suit!

As I began the healing, Polly was aware of my hands being intensely hot on her head and body and her emotions were starting to be released. As I moved down her body, I noticed that Polly had gone to "sleep". She had quieted, her breathing had altered and she looked serene and calm.

As we sat talking afterwards, Polly told me she had actually felt herself physically "lift" out of her body and "found" herself in a beautiful garden, full of flowers of every hue and description, but all the while aware of this constant feeling of hovering above the bed.

Polly was to leave with a sense of peace and a feeling of calm.

This strange phenomenon of falling to sleep had happened with all my clients and seemed to be part of the healing process, allowing them to go on and heal themselves.

I was to eventually call it their "Sacred Reiki Journey". I felt that this was a fitting name for their experiences as part of their Reiki treatment.

At 6.30am on Friday 7 July, I tripped and fell over cables lying on the floor at work, hurting my lower back and the top of my right arm. This accident would prove to be a life changing event for me and one that would prove, in time that it had been engineered by the Angels to get me out of work and do what I had been born to do; heal and teach!

On Tuesday 11 July, Doreen was operated on and the tumour was successfully removed, but two days later Gwen lost her fight against lung cancer and Doreen rang me to say that she had passed over with the biggest smile on her face.

We all felt that she had "hung on" long enough to see Doreen come through her operation safely and she could then pass over peacefully knowing Jock was waiting for her as she made her transition from this life to the next.

On Saturday 19 August, Polly rang to tell me that she had been back to the hospital the previous day to see her consultant and that he had given her the most wonderful news; her "aggressive cancer" had gone into remission.

Polly immediately booked a holiday to Majorca with her husband, son, daughter-in-law and grandchildren, which was wonderful news.

It was about this time Noel Edmunds was telling everyone about "The Cosmic Ordering Service" and how it had worked for him. You just asked the Cosmos for what you would like and if it was for your Highest and Greatest good, the prayer was answered! So, I thought that I would give it a try. After all I had nothing to lose!

Dear Cosmic Ordering Service,

I would like enough money to have a new car and to fulfil my dream of finishing work and becoming a full time Reiki Practitioner.

Thank you.

Margaret Ann Elson.

I then put this letter into an envelope under the bed and promptly forgot about it.

Saturday 16 September, Polly came back for a "top up healing". This was to be "mental and emotional healing" to help clear all the negative thoughts and emotions Polly had experienced whilst battling her condition.

On Monday 23 October, I now felt that at last I had achieved my destiny; Reiki Master at Teacher Level, although I still felt that "something" was missing. What? I had no idea, but Wendy Terry was to provide the answer.

On Wednesday 6 December, I arranged to meet Wendy Terry, who was quite well known locally for her Angel workshops and card readings.

I was to meet another kindred soul, Light Worker and Earth Angel.

We instantly clicked and sat chatting as if we had known each other for years.

Life was certainly getting better and at long last I was meeting like-minded people with whom I could connect on a spiritual level.

Wendy read the cards and told me that the Angels were asking me to finish work, enabling me to concentrate on Reiki fulltime. I told her there was no way I could finish work, because I just could not afford to do so. (The Angels had other plans; remember the fall I had at work in the July?)

At 4.30am on Thursday 7 December, as I stepped out of bed, I could vaguely see something on the floor next to the bed. Stooping down, I could see that it was a beautiful white feather. I just "knew" where it had come from. The Angels were showing themselves to me and this feather was proof of that. I instinctively knew that this was some kind of Angelic message yet to be revealed.

I picked the feather up and laughed and danced all around the bedroom like a madman, happy in the knowledge "they" had contacted me in this way.

Eight days later, "they" contacted me again, this time by phoning; yes phoning!

All God's angels come to us disguised

~ James Russell Lowell ~

At 6.00pm on Friday 15 December, the phone started to ring and it was displaying the numbers 1111111. Strange; what kind of number is that I thought as I answered it?

I kept repeating, "Hello?" but nobody answered. The line was totally dead. Putting the phone down, it immediately rang again; the same numbers and, once again, no one there! Two minutes later it rang again and for the third time the number was 1111111.

I picked the phone up, but did not speak. There was no sound, no connection; nothing at all. I put the phone down and determined that if it rang again I would not answer it as it was obviously someone playing the fool. It did not ring again that night. In fact it was the following March before "they" rang again.

2007

On Friday 12 January, whilst I was reading a book by Doreen Virtue, "Healing with the Angels", I saw the following passage:

"One of the ways the Angels will use to contact you is by showing you the numbers 1111."

I must have read the words over and over again until, at last, the penny dropped. The Angels had contacted me and they had done it by showing me feathers, numbers and by phoning! How exciting, yet who could I tell and, more to the point, who would believe me?

Paul Thomas; that's who!

On Friday 9 February, whilst walking out of a local supermarket, I heard my name being called. I turned around and there stood Paul Thomas. Paul and I had met at the Spiritualist Church when he came to sit in circle and recognition was instant for both of us. We were reconnecting on a soul level, going back to when we had walked together in past lives. Meeting him again was to be the start of the most amazing friendship, spanning thousands of miles.

Paul is now in Canada, but distance is no barrier, since we are connected to one another as if we were standing side by side. The Angels also connect to Paul, using feathers and numbers, especially 1111.

Paul is my spiritual soul mate and we both acknowledge that we walked together in many previous lives and, even more of a coincidence, Paul was also attuned to Reiki by Chris Ward! Definitely another Light worker/Earth Angel!

On Thursday 11 January, I acquired my (nearly) new car.

The previous Saturday, Pip had gone 'round to the local shop in our old car and whilst there someone had reversed into it, which badly dented the door and wing. They then drove away without telling us. This was such a shock and so upsetting that someone could do something like this and then not accept responsibility for their actions.

It was going to prove very expensive to repair and we just did not know what we were going to do, when a voice inside my head said, "New car. That's what you asked for so here it is."

Remember, I had asked the Cosmic Ordering Service for a new car in August 2006? Well, my plea had been heard and answered! They had listened to what I had asked for and barely five months later, a (nearly) new car!

At this time, Pip and Cheryl worked for a local garage and had picked out a car that they thought I would like. I totally ignored their choice and instead was guided to a car with VSP (Very Special Person) as part of the registration.

"That's the car for me," I said, much to the astonishment of Pip, Cheryl and the car salesman.

What did this episode teach me? Ask, believe, visualise and it will be yours. All I needed to do now was to visualise finishing work!!!

On Tuesday 13 March, Sally went for a scan to see how the tumour has reacted to the intense treatment that she had had to endure for the previous few months. I sat in meditation and linked in at the time she was due to have her scan.

I was utterly convinced that the result would come back with a resounding positive "all clear". (Sally was to say later that she actually saw me and her deceased granddad standing at the side of the scanning machine and she knew then that she would be given the all clear).

On Wednesday 14 March, I went back to see Wendy, again for an Angel Card reading and once again she told me that the Angels were requesting that I finished work. I still did not see how this would be possible financially.

At 3pm when I arrived home from visiting Wendy, the phone started ringing. It was another silent call with the same number as before. Confirmation from the Angels regarding what Wendy had told me that afternoon?

On the morning of Sunday 18 March, the strangest thing happened. As I sat in bed meditating, ectoplasm came and brushed against the bedroom window and then disappeared. I sat there staring at the bedroom window, totally baffled by what I had just seen.

The moment Cheryl walked into the bedroom "it" was there again!

"What the hell was that?" Cheryl ran to the window to see where "it" had gone.

We then looked at each other and said, "What on earth was that about?"

We both acknowledged that it was "Spirit" and that it was some kind of "message", but what the message was, we had no idea.

On Tuesday 20 March, Sally was given the most marvellous news. She had gone back to the hospital for her results from the scan to be told that she was in remission.

Who did she see standing at the back of the room once again? Her grandad and me of course!

On Thursday 3 May, I had my first student; First Degree Reiki. I was really excited and felt that at long last my dream was coming to fruition. I was nervous, but at the same time confident that it would be a learning curve for me.

Friday 29 June turned out to be my last day at work. Things had not been going well for me for quite some time and I was desperate to get out of having to go to work in such a negative place. I had been asking and praying every day for months that the Angels would get me out of there.... and fast!

I walked into work and just knew that I had had enough. I felt physically ill and broke down in tears.

I was subsequently diagnosed with reactive stress and depression and I was off work for the next two months.

On Tuesday 14 August, I held my second Reiki 1 workshop and this time I was really excited. I had received such a positive response from Wendy, my first Reiki student that I knew I was capable of dealing with what was being put there for me.

Teachers open the door, but you must enter.....by yourself

- Chinese Proverb -

On Saturday 18 August, Polly rang to tell me that she was still in remission from her cancer, one year on. I was overjoyed at this news and gave humble thanks to the Divine Source for the miracle that had taken place the year before.

On Friday 24 August, I decided to finish work. I handed in my notice and immediately felt a huge weight had been lifted from my shoulders. I was soon to realise why!

The accident and the angst that I was suffering were all part of the Master plan to get me to leave work. The Angels had used whatever means possible in helping me to achieve my destiny as a Reiki Master and teacher and, being at work, I could not give it the time and attention it warranted.

It is when we go against what we are being "told" that life becomes hard and quite often, as in my case, leaves us feeling physically and mentally drained. It was that simple. The lessons learnt from this are to go with your gut instinct, because it will never let you down.

On Saturday 6 October, whilst on holiday in Ibiza, we decided to go and visit the Cathedral in Ibiza Town. This is something we both like to do wherever we go on holiday and I always light a candle for Mum and Dad.

As I walked into the Cathedral, I went to sit on the left hand side, when a very loud, clear voice behind my left ear said, "No, not there! Over on the right".

I went and sat on the right hand side of the Cathedral, said my prayers and, as I opened my eyes, there on the floor in front of me was Rapid River's feather! He was there, right beside me, in Ibiza Cathedral.

This was so exciting and made me want to jump up and down with joy and whoop and holler at the top of my voice, but reasoning prevailed. I was in a place of worship after all.

At 10am on Friday 19 October, Doreen phoned and asked me if I could help with her daughter Collette who was five months' pregnant.

Doreen told me that Collette had been for a routine scan that morning and the hospital were concerned over the baby's failure to grow and also the apparent lack of a heart beat.

As I spoke with Doreen, I linked into Rapid River and he showed me the baby curled up, very comfortably and that "he" was alright.

At 11.30am, Collette was really upset at the thought that something was wrong with her baby, but as soon as I placed my hands over her abdomen, he gave one almighty kick, almost as if he was showing us that he did not like being disturbed. We both laughed out loud and we both knew from "his" actions that he was fine.

On Monday 12 November, *Mavis who had lost her husband *George in 2005, came for a Reiki treatment in the hope that it would help to reconcile her with the loss of her husband and the grief of losing her son in 2004.

Her daughter *Kelly, who was Collette's best friend, had treated her mum to a Reiki treatment on Collette's recommendation.

The healing for Mavis was both mental and emotional, with Mavis going on her Sacred Reiki Journey for an hour before I was allowed to call her back.

As we sat talking, her husband George came in carrying a bunch of Sweet Peas and told me they were for Mavis. He asked me to tell her that he had been watching as she planted Sweet Peas a few days before.

The look that came over Mavis's face was one of sheer disbelief. A couple of days before, Mavis had planted Sweet Peas given to her by her dad in memory of George.

Mavis took this message as proof that George was still with her and watching over her in the spiritual sense. Though Mavis found this a huge comfort, she would always miss his physical presence.

On Tuesday 11 December, *Mavis's daughter *Kelly came to see me.

Kelly was so emotionally traumatised by the loss of her dad and her brother that she felt helpless in coping with her own grief. She had seen how the Reiki had helped her Mum and Collette, so she had decided to try it for herself.

As we sat talking, her brother *Dean came in and showed me an image of them "fighting" over a spade whilst helping their dad with the gardening. Kelly remembered this and even started to laugh at the memory.

Dean also showed me a scene of them playing with a fort, a farm and of him pushing her in what looked like a Go-Kart.

Kelly confirmed all of this and remembered it vividly as they had been really close siblings.

Whilst channelling the energy through for Kelly, Dean showed me the "Messages from your Angels" cards by Doreen Virtue and asked me to ask Kelly about "Angels".

When I repeated to Kelly what Dean had said, she became very upset, crying uncontrollably for quite a few minutes before she was able to compose herself. Kelly was to tell me that the Robbie Williams' song "Angels" had been played at Dean's funeral and the year before, as she was giving birth, this song had come on the radio.

Kelly took this message as proof that Dean was still around watching over her and was greatly comforted.

The guardian angels of life fly so high as to be beyond our sight, but they are always looking down upon us

~ Jean Paul Richter ~

2008

On Saturday 9 January, I started to train as a Support Worker for Cruse Bereavement Charity to support people affected by the loss of a loved one. In doing this I felt that because of my past experiences I could empathise with people and try to help with their grief just by listening. All that is required is a small percentage of your time to sit and listen whilst the client's unload their burden of grief!

Unfortunately, it was a luxury that I never had when I lost mum, but a valuable lesson for me to be able to empathise with others who have been bereaved.

Doing the course brought me into contact with people that I had not seen in years and it was to be the start of new friendships.

On Wednesday 6 February, I received a text from Colleen to say that the baby was fine and everything was ok.

On Friday 3 March, a gentleman named *Barry had booked in for a healing.

Rapid River appeared in his business suit during my meditation and told me that it was going to be a very emotional, as well as a physical, healing for Barry.

Whilst using the pendulum over his energy centres, it showed me that his throat, heart and solar plexus chakras were all blocked with negative energy and a feeling that it had been lying their dormant for quite some time.

Imagine my surprise when laying my hands over his Heart and solar plexus I could "see" Barry dressed in a 14th century soldier's uniform, complete with breast plate, chain mail and sword. I immediately opened my eyes, more in shock, I think, than anything else.

I had never experienced anything like this before and of course when I looked at Barry he was dressed in modern day jeans and T shirt.

"Ok, just go with it," was my immediate thought.

I was then shown an arrow going into Barry's solar plexus and coming out on the top of his shoulder. As I placed my hands over the entry and exit wounds, the energy coming through my hands became very intense, with the feeling that I had my hands immersed in boiling water.

Afterwards, as we sat and discussed the healing, I asked Barry if he suffered from any discomfort in the area of his heart and solar plexus and also in the left shoulder region. Imagine my surprise when he said that for as long as he could remember he had had this lump on his shoulder and suffered huge discomfort in his midriff region, yet numerous medical tests had always come back negative.

I explained to him what I had experienced and told him that I thought all of his problems stemmed from his injuries sustained in a past life as a soldier. The lump and the pain in the midriff had all been brought forward from this past life.

I think Barry was as amazed as I was at what had transpired during the healing and could not quite believe what had happened.

On Friday 10 March, Barry called by to tell me that he had not felt that good in years and he believed that it was all down to the healing he had received the week before.

On Saturday 15 March, Doreen phoned to tell me that Collette had given birth to a healthy baby boy and that both mother and baby were fine.

At 1.30am on Wednesday 26 March, I was awoken from a deep sleep by the sound of someone sobbing as if their heart was broken.

I got out of bed and went and stood on the landing trying to work out where this sound was coming from. I felt really uneasy, with a deep sense of foreboding that something was terribly wrong. It was exactly the same feeling that I had experienced the night that Pip's dad had passed over. My gut instinct told me that it wasn't Grahame or Cheryl. However, I knew that it was a young soul crying out and I also knew that it was in spirit. I could not explain why; I just knew!

A voice behind my right ear told me to look at the clock, 1.30am and that all would be made clear later.

I got back into bed, eventually dropping off to sleep, but I was to wake up deeply troubled by what had occurred in the night.

At 10.00am on the Wednesday morning, I received a telephone call from *Sylvia, a lady who had been to see me for a Reiki treatment a few weeks before. Sylvia was asking if I could see her daughter *Mary that afternoon. She did not give me an explanation other than her daughter was desperately in need of help.

In meditation before Mary arrived, Rapid River was totally unforthcoming, which was strangely puzzling and very unusual for him.

At 1.00pm Mary arrived, accompanied by her mum. I have never ever seen a person so consumed with grief and utter despair. Her eyes were totally lifeless. The burden she was carrying was too huge for her small shoulders to carry and my heart immediately went out to her.

As I started to lay my hands on Mary, two things happened in quick succession; Rapid River was on my left side and a young man came and stood on my right.

It was the young man who had awoken me up in the night with his sobbing! This shook me and, if I am honest, frightened me as to where this was going.

"Trust!" That was the word that Rapid River whispered in my ear and that is what I did.

Channelling the healing over Mary's heart chakra, the intensity magnified and became so hot it was almost unbearable. Broken heart? That was the question that jumped into my mind, but Mary's defences were up and no one was going to penetrate this wall.

As I progressed with the healing, I began to feel as though my heart was broken and wanted to weep with her in her grief. It was so encompassing that it was penetrating my wall of protection. (I had not witnessed this before and it was a stark lesson for me in learning how to protect myself and my aura).

As Mary and I sat talking after the healing, *Henry came and stood beside his mum. He told me that he was Mary's son and he had been killed in a road accident a few months previously. Henry wanted me to tell his mum that he was sorry that he had had to leave like he did, but he wanted her to know that he was still around and watching over them.

If I am honest, I did not know what to do. It totally unnerved me as to how I was to approach his mum with this information and I knew that I had to handle it in a respectful and delicate way. One wrong word and the consequences would be horrendous.

Then, the strangest thing happened. It was as if I stepped out of my body and Henry stepped in and I stood there listening as he told his mum everything she needed to know.

I relayed the incident in the night to Mary; how I had been woken up and told to look at the clock. Mary confirmed that 1.30am was the time Henry had been killed. I was deeply shocked at this revelation.

Mary acknowledged that she had been asking for a sign from Henry to let her know that he was alright. She also admitted that she would never be able to get over this tragedy; that it would stay with her for the rest of her life.

One question that I still have is; did Henry know that his mum was coming to see me that day? I like to think so and that is why he "woke" me up at 1.30am.

On Thursday 16 October, I received an email from Eileen, a lady who lived and worked in Italy, asking me to send her some information on Reiki. At first I thought that it was some kind of joke, but I duly sent the relevant information.

Eileen emailed back asking if she could come on the 6 December and do a First Degree Reiki workshop with me! I had to pinch myself as I could not believe what was written in front of me and all the way from Italy!

On Friday 5 December, I was in my treatment room when I noticed a movement out of the corner of my eye. A beautiful butterfly was there in my Reiki room and I could not believe my eyes; after all it was December!

I was even more surprised when the butterfly "spoke" to me and said that he was Eileen's grandad in spirit and he wanted to introduce himself. He told me that he was very excited Eileen was coming there to do her Reiki and he had given her a message through a medium that I would be the one to teach her. My immediate thought was how could he recommend me when he did not even know me and he was in Spirit?

I also thought to myself that if anyone could hear me talking to a butterfly, they would definitely think that I had lost the plot!

At 9am on Saturday 6 December, I walked into my Reiki room to see if the butterfly was still there. I was really disappointed to find that it had disappeared. I had wanted to verify with Eileen what I had been told and now it was nowhere to be seen.

Eileen arrived at 9.30am and once again I immediately recognised a kindred soul. We chatted as if we had known one another for years and the dividing years made not a scrap of difference; we clicked!

At 12.30pm, I went down into the kitchen to prepare lunch and as I walked back into my Reiki room, Eileen was standing by the window talking to...... a butterfly.

"This is my grandad and it is through him that I am here today!"

My jaw just fell to the floor!

Eileen then explained that she had been thinking about doing a Complementary Therapy Course in Reflexology not Reiki. She had gone to see a Medium who gave her a message from her grandfather that she was not to do Reflexology; she was to do Reiki and the lady that would teach her would be shown to her.

Eileen said she felt quite confused by this message as Reiki had not even entered her mind.

Whilst browsing an American Angel website, my website came up. She felt that there was a connection, but still carried on looking just in case. Eileen then typed Reiki into the browser and there I was again at:

http://www.sacredreikijourney.co.uk

We spent a wonderful day together, Master and student, with Eileen proving to be a very astute student with the will and desire to heal in abundance.

2009

At 9.15am on Thursday 1 January, I asked for a message from the Angels just to let me know everything was as it should be.

At 12.00pm, I received an email from Eileen asking to come back and do her Reiki 2!

On Saturday 3 January, we booked our dream holiday; a Nile Cruise in Egypt. I was going home at last!

On Wednesday 7 January, I received a cheque for the injuries sustained from my accident at work and this verified what I had been told; that the Angels will help you in abundance, allowing you to do their work here without any financial worries.

On Tuesday 17 March, a gentleman named *Rod came to see me.

Once again, Rapid River was dressed in his power suit and showed me a "dark spot" in the lower bowel. This was confirmed by Rod before his treatment began.

The healing for Rod was extremely powerful and once again my hands felt as if they were immersed in boiling water. A lot of negative energy was released as tears for Rod's highest and greatest good.

He was to go on his Sacred Reiki Journey for an hour and was very reluctant to return to the present. He said that he had been "taken" to a place where he had found comfort, immense peace and felt so calm within himself he would have liked to stay there.

Before Rod left, I gave him a piece of paper with a positive affirmation printed on it: "I Deserve To Be Healed; I AM going to beat it" and asked him to say this Mantra morning, noon and night.

On Tuesday 26 March whilst in meditation, I became aware of a huge Red Indian standing in front of me. I knew instantly that it was not my guide Saskatchewan, but even so he had an important message for me. From that day onwards, I was to be known as Mags Wise Owl. This was the name I had been known as in a past life and one I should have again, confirming my wisdom and knowledge.

As he stood there telling me this, the love that abounded from him filled me with such emotion that I broke down in tears.

On Sunday 5 April, Jayne Hale, whom I had met at a "Goddess" workshop, did an Angel Card reading for me.

"The Angels are showing me that you should write a book. Go with the flow and see what happens. Write poetry, but definitely a book; it will be an inspiration to all who read it. Just tell it like it is, as if you are talking."

My immediate reaction to this message was "What on earth could I write about?" I hadn't a clue!

On Saturday 2 May, whilst channelling a healing, I was given the following message: "One minute past midnight, 5 October 1946, a Light Worker came to Earth".

I was "told" this was to be the first line of my book and to "Get on with it!"

A week later on Saturday 9 May, I was given the first line of Part Two: "He's here you know". These are Pip's words whenever he "smells" Dads tobacco.

***The act of putting pen to paper
encourages pause for thought.***

***This in turn makes us think more deeply about
life, which helps us regain our equilibrium***

~ Norbet Platt ~

On Thursday 14 May, we received a letter from the travel agent informing us that we had been upgraded to the Ms Mahrousa, a 5* Nile Cruise Ship. We were booked on a 3* and now we were being upgraded to a 5*?

I was extremely puzzled to why this should be, so I rang the travel agent for an explanation.

"There are not enough bookings to warrant the Ms *Seti sailing, so we have upgraded you. I hope that you do not mind?"

"Mind? You have got to be kidding me! Is this some kind of joke?"

The travel agent assured me that it was not a joke and that the Ms *Seti had been taken out of service as there were not enough passengers to warrant her sailing.

I was beside myself with excitement and could not believe what my gut instinct was telling me; that this was the work of the Angels and I was going to be sailing down the Nile on a 5* Cruise ship.

This holiday had been my dream for years and now I was going to be sailing in style. Perfect!

On Tuesday 19 May as I was packing for the Egyptian cruise, I was told to take my Fairy Cards, but I had no idea why.

On Wednesday 20 May, we flew to Egypt to live my dream. I knew that I was going home. After all, I had lived there in 680 BC.

At 7.30 pm, we were the first to arrive in the dining room and we were met with friendly smiles and made to feel very welcome by the staff.

Next to arrive were *Kay and *Ben who, when we introduced ourselves, said that they were also from the Midlands. *Graeme and *Jayne were next, followed by *Bryn and *Ali.

We all introduced ourselves and my gut feeling was that we had some really nice people on our table.

We were all chatting away when I noticed that Kay was very subdued, almost as if she had the worries of the world on her shoulders.

As we sat talking, a man in Spirit came and stood next to Bryn. He told me that he was Bryn's uncle and wanted him to know that he was there with him. I told him that he would have to wait for that, as I did not want to be thrown off the ship before my holiday had even begun!

Going down to our cabin later I stopped short and started laughing; the number on the cabin door opposite ours was 111.

At 7.00am on Thursday 21 May, we visited the Karnak and Luxor Temples.

As we stood in the reception waiting for our bus to arrive, Bryn hobbled up to us, accompanied by his wife Ali. I could see that they both looked upset and asked if there was a problem.

"Yes, it's my dratted feet and ankles," said Bryn and then went on to explain how the day before they were due to fly out to Egypt, Bryn's feet and ankles had swollen up and he was now having difficulty walking. Bryn knew that he would not be able to accompany Ali walking around the temples, as it would be far too uncomfortable. Just a few steps were difficult, so he was going to have to stop on board whilst we all went off and enjoyed ourselves and, naturally Bryn was really unhappy about this.

I took Bryn to one side and offered to do Reiki on him. His reply took me by surprise.

"No thanks. I've met your sort before" and turning walked away leaving me with the thought;

"That'll teach you to poke your nose in where it's not wanted,"

So off we went to visit the temples minus Bryn, taking Ali with us in our group. On our way, our guide Abdul was explaining about Egyptian hieroglyphics and asked if anyone had the initial M as their first name. I put my hand up and his next words astounded me. In Egyptian hieroglyphics I would be known as Wise Owl; confirmation once more, if needed!

I had only been there two days and already I had seen 111 and now Abdul was confirming what I had been told by my Spirit Indian. Whatever is going to happen next?

At 11.00am on the way back to the ship, we called at a perfumery factory in the middle of Luxor. We were shown demonstrations of how perfume is made and then we could buy whatever we wanted.

Pip and I wandered off to a part of the factory that nobody else seemed interested in, when one of the guides came up to me and told me that I had dropped a £100.00 Egyptian note. I was totally baffled by this, because at this stage I had not had my purse out, but Ahab insisted that it was mine as he had seen it drop out of my purse. "Okay," I thought, "go with it". Obviously someone in our group had dropped it.

At 2.00pm, sitting in the lounge back on board ship, Graeme and Jayne came and sat next to us and started talking. Graeme said that he was upset because he had lost a £100.00 Egyptian note that morning and could not think where. The only place that he could think of was the perfumery factory.

The look on Graeme's face when I told him what had happened and said that I had been waiting for someone to say that they had lost £100 Egyptian note, was one of sheer amazement. He thought that he had lost it for good and that was it. Never for one minute did he think that he would end up sitting next to the person who had been given it.

Ahab could have so easily pocketed that money and no one would have been any the wiser. This proved to me that there are still honest people out there and it helps to restores your faith in human nature.

At 3.00pm sitting up on deck enjoying the sights and sounds of Luxor, Kay and Ben came and asked if they could sit with us.

"I came to Tutbury Castle and had a Tarot card reading," said Kay, out of the blue!

Pip immediately said, "Oh! Marg does that."

Kay then asked if I had my cards with me and, if so, would I mind doing a reading for her? (Now I understood why I had been told to pack my cards).

As I shuffled the cards, a little old lady came and stood next to Kay. I knew instantly that she was still here on the earth plane. When I described this lady to Kay, she became really upset and said that it was a description of her beloved Nana who had been battling Alzheimer's for nearly two years. Nana had not spoken or recognised Kay for this length of time and this was hurting Kay very much.

Nana then asked me to give the name "Peter" to Kay and this was met with floods of tears. Peter was the name that Nana used to describe whatever she looked at.

The reading and giving her the messages from her beloved Nana proved to be so beneficial to Kay that she said she felt better than she had in a long time.

At 7.30pm, Kay walked into the dining room that night with the biggest smile on her face and, when questioned, she said that it was down to the messages I had given her that afternoon.

Bryn again made the comment, "Yes I've met her sort before. Don't believe everything they tell you."

This remark was met with total silence by the rest of the table and poor Ali looked really embarrassed.

At 9.00pm, sitting in the lounge bar on my own, Bryn walked in and asked if the offer of Reiki still stood.

I was quite shocked by his question and thought at first he was joking, but by the look on his face I knew that it had taken a lot of courage for him to ask me.

As we sat talking, I put my hand on his shoulder and mentally asked the Reiki to flow for Bryn's highest and greatest good. Bryn was taken aback that this was all you had to do to get Reiki to flow. Bryn then opened his heart and proceeded to tell me of his childhood with his "spiritual healer" Dad; hence the remark he had made to me.

These events from Bryn's upbringing had incurred manifestation in the form of physical ailments, heart attack, stroke and the day before coming on holiday to Egypt, as he had already told me, his feet and ankles had blown up out of all proportion.

I told him that I had seen his uncle standing by his side on the first night in the dining room, even describing him in minute detail and told him that he wanted Bryn to know he was there. It turned out Uncle *Patrick had been more of a dad to him than his own flesh and blood and my heart went out to him at this revelation.

As Bryn was talking, his hurt and anger became obvious. This towering rage inside of him that had been there ever since he could remember and poor Ali was getting the brunt of it.

I questioned him; "If you know are upsetting Ali by your behaviour, why persist in doing it?"

It was obvious to all that Ali was visibly upset at his remark to me earlier in the evening and was embarrassed by his behaviour.

By this stage, Bryn was on the verge of tears and I felt that underneath all this bravado was a little boy who so desperately wanted to be loved, but at the same time felt he had to put up a front so that he did not get "hurt". Bryn agreed with me that this was the case and stopped him from getting hurt, but did it? That was my question to Bryn. His reply was, "No, because I know that I am hurting Ali with my behaviour."

After talking for what seemed like days and giving him Reiki, Bryn said that he felt "different", calm even; something he had not felt in years.

Bryn was now 66-years-old and his abrasive childhood was still having an effect on his health today.

Our childhood and upbringing has such a monumental affect on our adulthood and unless we can address these issues, deal with them and move on, they can manifest into a physical/psychological problem.

It is never too late to have a happy childhood

~Tom Robbins~

At 7.00am on Friday 22 May, we visited the Valley of the Kings and the Valley of the Queens in Luxor on the West Bank.

Bryn accompanied us. His swollen feet and ankles had gone down and even though they were still slightly sore, he had managed to get his boots on and he walked all morning without any trouble.

By 8.00am, we were at The Valley of the Kings on the West bank of the Nile. It was a magnificent Burial Ground for the Pharaohs and was also known as the Kingdom of Osiris, God of the underworld where the Pharaohs met their Gods. Their grand tombs where the Egyptian Pharaohs believed they would embark on a journey in which they would meet the gods in the afterlife were filled with treasures and beautiful artefacts as payment to the Gods to achieve immortality.

As we walked into the Valley of the Kings, the heat was so intense, but all around me I could feel watching eyes. The feeling of being in such a sacred place was immense and, even though there were hundreds of tourists around, you could still feel the reverence of the place.

Going down into the different tombs was intensely moving. The hieroglyphic drawings, with their amazing colours as fresh today as they were thousands of years ago, have to be seen to be believed!

At 10.00am we arrived at the Valley of the Queens, which is also located on the West bank of the Nile. As we drove up to Queen Hatshepsut's Funerary Temple, I was overcome with the most powerful of emotions and I broke down in floods of tears. I was home! My gut instinct told me I had been there before in a former life, in what kind of discipline I had no idea. I had a sense of belonging that I had not perceived when we were in the Valley of the Kings.

As I walked around this Temple, I could feel Queen Hatshepsut's presence by my side, almost as though she were giving me a guided tour of her own.

I felt very sad when the time came to leave, but I said my goodbyes to her and told her that one day I would be back and that we would meet again.

At 2.00pm on Friday, our boat set sail for Edfu and its Temple of Horus. Sailing down the Nile with the sights and sounds of a bygone era passing by, Jayne came across and nervously asked me if I would do a reading for her.

As I shuffled the cards, I was told that there was a problem in her working life and this problem was making life hard to cope with. Jayne confirmed this. I was given the message that she had nothing to worry about, that all was being taken care of and "they" were more than aware of what problems this person was creating.

I was then shown the letter C and told that this was the first initial of the person involved. Jayne was taken aback by this information but confirmed it was *Coral. At that precise moment, a ship going back up the Nile hooted at our boat as it passed by. We both turned to look and there on the side of the ship was the name "Coral". This confirmation led us both to burst out laughing.

Once more the Angels were showing us that they had been listening and the name on the side of the ship was confirmation.

On Saturday 23 May, we visited the High Dam in Aswan and on the way back to Luxor we called at a Papyrus Institute.

Whilst gazing at the papyrus pictures, I felt a tap on my arm. Turning around, a young Egyptian man was standing beside me with a huge smile on his face.

"You have the smile of Nefertiti" he said and he then turned and walked away, leaving me feeling totally perplexed by his comment.

It was some time later after this visit that I realised I had been drawn to purchase a bust of Queen Nefertiti at the Alabaster factory in Luxor on only our second day there in Egypt.

At 1.00pm, walking back on board ship, Kay was waiting to meet me and I could tell by looking at her that she was buzzing with excitement.

As I walked up to her, she thrust her left hand out for me to look; on her third finger sat the most exquisite engagement ring. Kay and Ben had decided that morning to go into Aswan, buy a ring and get engaged.

We hugged and danced together. I was so thrilled for them both.

I made my excuses and went to find Abdul to try and arrange a cake for this most auspicious of occasions. Abdul was just as delighted and said, "Leave everything to me; I will sort it all".

At 7.30pm in the Dining Room, I was sat at the dining room table grinning like the cat that had got the cream. I knew what was coming!

Once everyone had had their dinner, the crew came out of the kitchen with Abdul leading, holding a beautiful cake. One of the crew members was playing a drum and the others were all making a keening sound.

Kay was confused as to what was happening. Then, as Abdul walked up to her she turned to me and said, "This is your doing isn't it?"

Abdul then got Kay and Ben to stand in the middle of the dining room and we all circled around them waving our serviettes. It was fabulous and, what a memory, not only for Kay and Ben but for the rest of us; something we would not forget in a hurry.

I have to say a big thank you to Abdul and the crew for making such an effort in ensuring that Ben and Kay would never forget their engagement day.

On Sunday 24 May, we visited the Botanical Gardens in Aswan and from here you can look over to the Aga Khans mausoleum situated on the West bank of the Nile, overlooking the Monastery of St. Simeons.

We sailed back from Elephantine Island to our boat on a Felucca, just like in Biblical times. Magical!

On Monday 25 May, we had to get up at 3.00am to travel south to Aswan, close to the border with Sudan, to visit the site of Ramses II and Queen Nefertiti at Abu Simbel.

As you walk up to this site, the image that greets you is breathtaking in its splendour and majesty. The colossal figures of Ramses II and Queen Nefertiti is a sight that literally takes your breath away and you gaze in awe and wonder at how they were able to achieve such magnificence all those centuries ago!

The inner temple is so precisely oriented that twice every year on 22nd February and 22nd October, the first rays of the morning sun shine down the entire length of the inner temple, illuminating the back wall of the innermost shrine and the statues of the four gods seated there; Ptah, Amun-Ra, Ramses II and Re-Horakhte.

Ptah is the primal creator, the first of all the gods, creator of the world and all that is in it. He is not created, but simply is.

Amun-Ra is believed to be the physical father of all Pharaohs, King of the Gods of Egypt and Patron of the Pharaohs.

Ramses II (reigned1304-1237 BC) was the third ruler of the Nineteenth Dynasty of Egypt. A great warrior, he was also the builder of some of Egypt's most famous monuments.

Re-Horakhte, Re (Ra) was the Egyptian sun god who was also often referred to as Re-Horakhty, meaning Re (is) Horus of the Horizon, referring to the god's character. The early Egyptians believed that he created the world and the rising sun was, for them, the symbol of creation. The daily cycle, as the sun rose, then set only to rise again the next morning, symbolised renewal and so Re was seen as the paramount force of creation.

At 1.00 pm, we were back on board ship and started sailing back up to Luxor that afternoon. It signalled the beginning of our journey back home and, naturally, everyone was feeling slightly downbeat.

My most outstanding memory from the holiday was of the wonderful Egyptian people; their friendliness and hospitality was second to none. Their spirituality was so inspiring and one that we as Europeans could learn from. They have nothing, yet they want for nothing.

My visit to Queen Hatshepsut's Temple will live with me forever and Ramses II Temple at Abu Simbel was awe inspiring!

Regarding the Karnak and Luxor temples, I feel humbled and privileged to have walked where Pharaohs once walked and worshipped.

The trip was what dreams are made of; sailing down the Nile whilst dining, biblical scenes floating by the window and last but not least the lovely people that I met on board ship.

Bryn and Ali had booked their holiday with the Ms Mahrousa, whereas Graeme, Jayne, Ben and Kay, like us, had also been upgraded. So, was this all part of the Master plan? Who knows!

On Tuesday 26 May, we were back in Luxor. As we sat talking on the top deck, a smaller boat came and docked alongside us. I looked at the name "Seti" and realised that this was the boat that we should have been on originally. When I enquired as to why the *Seti was now berthed beside us, I was told that it had been taken out of commission for a week and Tracy (rep) could give no logical explanation to what I had been told by the travel agent!

I had to smile to myself. What was this telling me?

On Wednesday 27 May, we flew back home and I felt really melancholy. I wanted to stop there; it was where I belonged, yet I had to go back 'home' to England.

At 9.30pm, we landed at Manchester airport. It was raining, cold and miserable. I felt that the weather matched how I was feeling inside and I longed to be back in my beautiful Egypt.

As we were waiting for the cases, Bryn came and shook my hand and thanked me for giving him Reiki and helping him in a way that he had not been helped before.

In Bryn's words "You will never know how much you helped me". With that, we had a big hug and he was gone. I was deeply touched and honoured at his remarks to me and also with a sense of pride that I had been able to reach out and help him in the way that he needed to be helped.

It is a wonderful gift to have been given; the ability to help people just by talking and I respect and honour every minute of it.

At 6am on Thursday 28 May, back home to normality! The washing machine was on and there were cases to unpack, yet all I wanted to do was to daydream and picture myself back in Egypt sailing down the Nile and reliving all of the magical things that we had seen and experienced.

I was suddenly awakened out of my dream state by Pip shouting from upstairs; something about "On the window".

I ran back upstairs and on our bedroom window was the shape of ISIS! We both just stood there staring at what was clearly the outline figure of Isis, Mother of the Nile. We were both too shocked to speak and could not comprehend how this figure could be on our window. We knew that we weren't imagining it, for it was clearly there in front of us.

At 9.00am, we asked Mick and Val, our next door neighbours, to come round and look at this "phenomenon" that had appeared on our bedroom window. They have kept birds for years and we thought they may have a logical explanation to how "ISIS" came to be on our window. They hadn't!

The very next morning Mick shouted for us to go 'round to their house urgently. On their conservatory window was the shape of ISIS, exactly as it had appeared on our window.

We were all completely mystified as to how this strange "outline" had materialised on our respective windows.

I tried to take a photograph of ISIS without success. It was as though "she" did not want to be photographed, but was for our eyes only.

Invocation of Isis

I, Isis, am all that hath been that is or shall be,

***I, who made light from my feathers,
the wind from my wings,***

No mortal man ever hath me unveiled!

- Until now -

So, this is my life story up to the point of publication. I have written it exactly as the Angels asked me to; as if I were talking. Sally, Doreen and Polly are enjoying life to the full. Rod is still having ongoing treatment, but is remaining upbeat, steadfast and strong.

Kay and Ben still keep in touch.

Whenever I go to visit Edna, the door bell will ring as we sit talking, but no one is ever there! We both acknowledge that it is Gary playing games and letting us know that he is still around.

I have a wonderful Reiki meditation circle with a group of ladies who are eager to learn about connecting with Source.

Pip is also awakening to Spirit, at long last! He is now noticing numbers, feathers and different kind of signs and this makes my heart sing.

I give thanks everyday for his unending love for me and I feel truly honoured and blessed to have this man by my side. He is my Twin Flame and I could not do what I have been born to do without his neverending support, sound advice and also in helping to keep me "grounded".

Having been on the threshold of taking my own life and knowing the utter despair that I was feeling of not being able to see my way forward, I am filled with great sadness whenever I hear the naive and callous comment, "They are selfish for doing that". There, but for the Grace of God go all of us!

Thank goodness I had a wonderful, understanding doctor and also my neighbour at the time, dear Tommy Neal, without whose intervention, I would not be telling my story now.

***Ignorance is the night of the mind, but
a night without a moon or star***

- Confucius -

That was the end of my book, or so I thought, until I received the following email from Angela Hickman, (author of the Book of Grace/Vol I: The Lost Pages) in response to me asking her to write the foreword to this book.

December 2009

Email from Angela Hickman:

Hi Mags,

I have just read your book with the view to writing the Foreword straight afterwards. As I was reading, I was getting this growing feeling that it wasn't finished. What I am getting is going against your feelings of getting it published, but I have to tell you what I'm getting then you can make up your own mind!

Firstly, I love the way you have written it - it is very easy to understand and I kept seeing a subtitle on it, "If I can do it……" I realised why later.

Rapid River came in to me as I got nearer to the end, along with Archangel Michael, Jesus and God (so if I don't tell you what they've shown me I'll get struck down with lightening!)

Rapid River showed me that all the healing stuff you do is, as yet, untapped and written. You have SO much more to offer to the world on top of this.

I got the strong feeling that what you have written is part 1 and you now need to explain about Reiki in your own simplistic terms…how it is.

Jesus will "channel" for you what needs to be written and how.

Your book will become a module for others to read and understand that Reiki is there for everyone. If I can do it then so can you!

That is the message that you will be sending out to all Light Workers waiting to be called to arms……and Reiki.

Love

Angela x

As I live each day may I do my part!
To make one difference, to touch one heart,
And through each day may it be my goal
To encourage one mind and inspire one soul!

www.friendsinneed.com/quotes.

Angela Hickman

I first met Angela at a "Holistic meet" in November 2006 where she was giving a talk on Angels. At this time I had never met Angela and did not know anything about her, other than she read Angel cards.

Later on in the evening, Angela gave everyone a pack of Angel cards with the intention that we gave each other a "reading".

Paul Thomas, who had invited me to go to this meeting, was sitting next to me and asked if I would "do" a reading for him with the Doreen Virtue Archangel cards. I was told to let Paul hold the cards and one specific card would then appear out of the pack, pertinent to him.

I was also given the words "Albert" and "wheat fields", which to me was puzzling and did not make one iota of sense.

The card bearing the words "Career Transition" came out of the pack and when I told Paul the words I had been given, he immediately began to laugh out loud. He told me that he was hoping to emigrate to Canada the following August if everything went to plan, hence the card "Career

Transition" and the words "Albert" and "wheat fields", since Alberta is the area where there are wheat fields in abundance.

I was amazed by this reading, but it was to prove that it was only the beginning of a gift that was to get stronger the more that I became connected to Reiki.

In December 2006, I was to meet Angela again at a Reiki share organised by Paul Thomas at our local Town Hall. Paul organised us into groups of threes; one "giving" one receiving and one person watching.

Paul asked if I would "give" to *Rhoda with Angela sitting in front watching. As I began to channel I was aware of a "Bright White Light" surrounding me, so bright in fact, it made me want to put my hands over my eyes to shield them, exactly as had happened when I sat on the rostrum at church.

Afterwards, I went and sat back down in my seat, only to find Angela sitting down next to me. Her next question left me speechless.

"Do you realise that you work with Jesus?"

I looked at her blankly, at the same time thinking, "How can I answer a question like that?" and not sound conceited.

"Well, it would nice to think so," I said, feeling myself blushing with embarrassment.

Angela then explained that she had "seen" Jesus standing with me as I was channelling Reiki for Rhoda, hence the "white light". I was totally taken aback by her words and could not quite believe what she had just told me but, oh boy, did I want it to be true.

I was to meet Angela again in June 2009. She came to my house and, as she walked in the front door she said, "Now I understand why I felt the "Christ Energy" when I connected to you" and promptly recalled our meeting at the Reiki share in December 2006.

Angela came to give me a very profound message that day and has continued to do so ever since and I salute her for the true messenger that she is.

Angela's book, channelled through her by Archangel Michael, is a must read for anyone starting out on their Spiritual pathway. As you begin to read this book, it resonates in your deepest soul to a time when we as Light Workers all walked the earth plane with our beloved Master, Jesus.

I have to admit that after reading Angela's advice and also speaking to her on the phone, my thoughts were in turmoil. What on earth would I be able to write about?

The following week, as I was meditating, these profound words were given to me:

And so to Reiki, Divine Source and The Angelic Realm....A Divine Explanation!

Trust only movement.

Life happens at the level of events, not of words.

Trust movement

- Alfred Adler -

Part Three

Reiki, Divine Source & The Angelic Realm

A Divinely Timed Message from "Angelic Gateways", Courtesy of Angela Hickman

Mags,
I channelled a message from Jesus for you under the posting: "Christmas Message Delivery" on the main wall on Xmas day - you might want to take a look :-)
Lots of Love
Angela x

Hi Mags,
Message from Jesus for you:
"The kindness of your heart can be felt by all those around you. Through your words you shall touch an ever wider audience and bring hope, comfort and most of all inspiring love to those whose eyes shall be cast upon them.

You feel my loving hand upon your shoulder, my words whispered in your ear and my fingers guiding your pen.

As it was my mission to bring love to this world, so it is yours blessed soul.

Namaste I AM Jesus, the Christ"

Jesus has guided my "pen" and below is the information needed to bring Light Workers~ Earth Angels into being.

To pick up the banner and go forth and heal and teach as you were meant to do from the day you were born!

It has been written for all those "lost souls" who are not quite sure why they are here and to what their purpose is at this momentous moment in time.

> ***I don't know what your destiny will be, but one thing I do know: the only ones among you who will be really happy are those who have sought and found how to serve***
>
> *~ **Schweitz**er, Albert ~*

Reiki: A Divine Explanation

Hands are the heart's landscape

~ ***Pope John** Paul II* ~

Reiki is the ancient art of "Laying on of Hands" in order to heal.

Reiki (pronounced Ray-Key) is a combination of two Japanese words, Rei and Ki, meaning "universal life energy".

To me, Reiki is a gift given by the Divine Source and I honour and respect it with the acknowledgement it deserves. Reiki is not to be used or abused flippantly.

Reiki is a powerful tool in helping to heal your fellow mankind and Mother Earth.

Remember back to your childhood when as a child the touch of your mother's hand soothed you when you needed comforting. A maternal instinct that was so strong for her child knowing just where you needed it, making it all go away and leaving you feeling safe and secure in the knowledge that you were loved, wanted and cared for.

That is Reiki at its most powerful and it has been given down the centuries without thought or recognition for what is basically a powerful tool for healing….our hands.

Touch is a means of communication without words and can convey a feeling of love to pass from one human being to another. This also includes animals when by touch a cat will purr and a dog will wag its tail in recognition of the hand laid upon them.

Research has shown that adults who were rarely touched in their formative years are more likely to suffer from depression, mental issues and social disorders; hardly surprising when touch is the most valuable source for healing.

Whilst Reiki is spiritual in nature, it is not a religion, has no dogma and is not dependent on what your beliefs are or not and you do not have to believe for it to work.

To be kind and compassionate, with a generous amount of empathy, reaching out with a loving heart and mind and not expecting anything in return does not make you "religious". These are the qualities needed to make you a conduit for Reiki Divine Source Healing energy. It's that simple.

There have been many arguments and wars down the centuries over religion in all its basic forms and, remember, Jesus was crucified for his beliefs.

Look at our modern world today; little has changed. Wars are still being fought in the name of religion. People are still being bombed, murdered and maimed and all for what? Power! That is what all wars have ever been about; Man's unachievable aim for world dominance.

Even when this so called "autonomous power" is realised, they will still not have the satisfaction they crave, ultimately leading them in their totally deluded state of mind to carry on with their unjustified killing and maiming.

Inciting and brainwashing others to kill and maim just because we do not share their beliefs and becoming in their eyes the enemy? How sad and disillusioned is that? We are all children of God regardless of colour, race or creed. Whatever you want to call the "Higher" energy, we are all still as one in Gods eyes.

You do not have to be religious to be spiritual and this is where Reiki comes into being. Reiki is unconditional love for your fellow man. It is universal with no strings attached, the ability to love and be loved in return, as sung by the late great Nat King Cole.

When Jesus walked the Earth plane healing and teaching, he was subjected to ongoing abuse, but with a quiet dignity he carried on regardless to what was said or thought about him. It is my belief that we as Light workers at this moment in time are here to spread this message to the world, to carry on what Jesus and his disciples started.

We are in service to the Divine and I am extremely humbled at the fact that Margaret Ann Elson has been chosen to help do his work in this lifetime, "healing and teaching" my fellow man.

Reiki is there for anyone who can give and most importantly "receive" love, encompassing the will to serve and the desire to heal.

Whether you are a rich man, poor man, a beggar man or a thief, Reiki is there for you. It's that simple and all that is required of you is to be a willing student capable of giving and receiving love.

Life is not about material gain. Being materialistic does not bring you the happiness and fulfilment that each and every one of us deserves. The state of the world at the present time is testament to that.

Everyone is suffering through man's greed of wanting more with the outcome being job losses, bankruptcy, homelessness, and destitution with a prevailing sense of not knowing where to go to find comfort!

Those poor souls who have seen no way out of their financial problems have been driven to take their own lives and all for what? A materialistic world where man has forgotten how to help his fellow man, how sad is that?

I grew up in a world that was recovering from a world war, where everything was rationed; food, clothing, etc. We lived in a three bedroom terrace with an outside toilet and no bathroom. Friday night was bath night; as a small child in the "copper" in the corner of the kitchen and then as I grew bigger, a tin bath brought from outside.

Remember, at this time there was no such thing as central heating. In wintertime it was freezing and I hated bath night with a vengeance!

I can remember having holes in my shoes with cardboard stuffed in the bottom to try and stop my feet from getting wet. I remember Mum apologising for not being able to buy me a new pair of shoes, sitting with her "empty" purse in the middle of the week and crying because she did not know how she was going to feed, clothe and keep us warm through winter.

I remember the windows being so thick with ice that you could not see through them and cuddling down in my bed and not daring to stick my nose above the cover for fear of frostbite. I had at least four blankets, an eiderdown and an army coat on top of me, with the weight making me feel that it was pushing me through the mattress.

We had "Lino" on the floor, which literally froze your bare feet as you stepped out of bed onto it and then, a little square of carpet to stand on, which to me at that time was sheer luxury.

In later years, we were to have fitted carpets throughout the house and instead of a dolly tub and copper Dad bought me a washing machine with a spinner attached. That was such a scary piece of machinery and I used to watch from afar as this "thing" used to jump and thrash about the kitchen like some demented animal!

The strange thing is that when reflecting on all of these memories, I cannot ever recall going hungry. I have a vision of this huge stew pot on the table filled with pork bones and loads of vegetables picked from our own garden.

(Pork bones; I have to smile when I see "pork bones" classed as "spare ribs" today in supermarkets and are classed as a "must have" on a Chinese takeaway!)

We had potatoes from our garden that were cooked in the ashes under the coal fire. The smell alone used to make your tummy "rumble" and, when cooked, if we were lucky a small knob of Red Seal margarine to put in them.

Chicken was a luxury you had once a year at Christmas. If not, you may have had pigs' brains, sheep's heart or some other disgusting offal.

Every year Mum used to buy me a new dress and a pair of shoes for the Sunday School Anniversary Concert. Oh boy, did I love this! All the girls used to swagger around like peacocks showing off their new dresses and shoes. The shoes had to last until the next year, in which time your feet would have grown so much that your poor toes would be scrunched up painfully and you had difficulty walking.

A consequence of wearing those ill-fitting shoes is hammer toes, from which I still suffer to this day.

I can remember cutting the toe out of my school pumps so that I would be able to run faster without my toes hurting me. I loved school; anything to do with sport and I was happy.

As for clothes; I have a school photograph of me wearing a cardigan that had more darns and holes than material, but what the heck. Everyone was in the same boat then so what did it matter?

I loved "chapel" and I used to go twice a day; Sunday school in the afternoon and then back with Mum and Dad at night.

Everybody seemed to "like" everyone else then; it was as if we were an extended family and to sing those wonderful hymns was a never ending joy to me.

Another memory I can recall is of not locking the door when we went out; no point when there was nothing to pinch. People respected each other and their properties then and harboured a genuine desire to help each other in their hour of need.

Our next door neighbour used to go out to work and Mum would go in and help polish and scrub floors on her hands and knees, and all without asking.

We all have to try and get back to these times and we can if we all pull together. This is where we as Light Workers come into being. We are here to teach everyone how a little bit of faith and positive thinking can go a long way; to teach man how to love not only himself but his fellow man and the abundance that can come from showing that we care about each other. It is our job to teach respect and kindness and the way we do that is by Reiki.

Each and every one of us has to come back to our Spiritual pathway and encompass into our beings all the love and abundance that is waiting there for us and us alone.

Dr Mikao Usui, our founder Father of Reiki, wrote the following five principles, hoping that every student would incorporate them into their lives:

- **Just for today do not worry**; God give me the strength to accept the things I cannot change, the courage to change the things I can and the wisdom to know the difference
- **Just for today do not anger;** Anger is a reaction; the response is LOVE
- **Honour your Parents, Teachers and Elders;** Remember our greatest teachers can be our students or a stranger in the street
- **Earn your living honestly**; Be true to yourself whatever your gift; acknowledge it, share it and rejoice in it
- **Show gratitude to every living thing;** It touches our heart centre when someone shows gratitude for something we have done. Remember to do the same!

A History of Reiki and its Founder, Dr Mikao Usui

(15 August 1865 – 9 March 1926)

Reiki originates from India and the Far East, dating back many thousands of years to the time before Jesus and Buddha.

The techniques were passed down through the ages by word of mouth, but unfortunately the techniques became diluted over the centuries until they were eventually lost.

Dr Usui, Principal of the Doshish University in Kyoto, Japan, was asked by one of his students if he could authenticate the healing by "laying on of hands" described in the Bible as an act of the Christ, Jesus. Dr. Usui replied that even though he was a Christian preacher and missionary he could not verify this fact.

Acting on this question, Dr Usui resigned from his position at the Doshish University and travelled to the University of Chicago in the United States with the hope and belief that in time he would be able to learn this healing skill described in the Bible.

After studying for several years, becoming a Doctor of Theology and not finding the answer to the question he sought, Dr Usui turned to other philosophies and religions and began to study Hinduism, Zoroastrianism[2] and Buddhism among others.

In Buddhist texts, he was to find information relating to the Buddha healing by "Laying on of hands" and he decided to return to a Buddhist temple located in Kyoto, Japan to carry on studying.

After many months he had still not found the information he so desperately sought relating to this phenomenon as told in the Bible. Realising that he needed to expand his search, he went to study in China, but once again did not find the answers that he was seeking.

Realising that many of the original Buddhist texts were written in Sanskrit, Dr Usui decided to learn this ancient language of India, eventually finding an inscription written in Sanskrit with the explanation of how to do the "Laying on of hands" healing.

Dr. Usui decided to return to Kyoto and talk to his mentor the senior monk of the Zen temple, about how to activate the energy he felt was needed to bring this phenomenon into being.

It was decided between them that Dr. Usui would go and meditate at the top of a nearby mountain - Mount Koriyama - a mountain known as an excellent place for meditation.

Dr Usui would go through this meditation without food - only water for 21 days in the hope that he would be

---

[2] Zoroastrianism is an ancient religion founded by the Persian prophet Zoroaster, the principal belief of which is in a supreme deity and a cosmic contest between two spirits, one good and one evil.

given the extra information he had been seeking for so many years. On the twenty first day, Dr. Usui had a spectacular "White Light" experience showing him how to activate the Divine Source Reiki energy symbols, enabling the healing known as "Laying on of hands".

After returning to a normal state of consciousness, Dr Usui began to climb down the mountain and in his rush he stumbled and injured his toe. He held his toe in his hands for a few minutes, the bleeding stopped and the pain disappeared.

Reaching the bottom of the mountain, he went to an inn and ordered a large meal. After fasting for so long he was warned about eating such a big meal. Nevertheless, he ate the meal without suffering any major consequences.

As he was sitting eating, Dr Usui noticed that the innkeeper's daughter's face was very swollen and she seemed to be in a lot of discomfort. After diagnosing her with a tooth abscess, Dr Usui laid his hands upon her face and within minutes the swelling and pain disappeared.

This was to be the start of the Usui system of Reiki Divine Source Energy Healing.

Dr Usui returned to his monastery, but after a few weeks decided to go to the slum quarters of Kyoto with the intention of teaching the beggars who lived there how to lead a better life. After several years treating various ailments and diseases, he began to notice that the same faces kept appearing all the time. When questioned, the beggars said that it was too troublesome working; it was far easier to carry on begging!!

Dr Usui was deeply shaken by this. He recognised that he had forgotten something of great importance; the principals for Holistic Healing.

Heal the Spirit, Heal the Body, Need for Gratitude. These are lessons that we all need to take on board. It is all too easy when you first start your Holistic pathway to want to "give" Reiki for free and I have learned the hard way that Reiki is not mine to give away.

In respect for the gift that you have been given there has to be an "energy" exchange and not necessarily monetary!

Reiki is My Life

Reiki is my life. I live, breathe, eat, and sleep it! I am so passionate about Reiki that I want to share it with the world and the only way I can do that is by writing a book about my life with an explanation as to how I became a Reiki Master at Teacher level.

Margaret Ann Elson, from humble beginnings, became a Reiki Master/Teacher. Whoever would have believed it? Definitely not me!

I want each and every one of you to find what I have found through Reiki. Anyone with the capacity to give and receive love is more than capable of becoming a Reiki Master; it is that simple. It is not a science; there are no "exams". All you have to do is put your trust in the Divine Source and the world is yours.

Since becoming a Reiki Master/Teacher, I have met various people who have told me they did not "feel" a connection when being attuned to Reiki. If this is the case, then we have to question the Master's intentions when attuning a student, be it First, Second or Master degree.

I would also call into question the Ego of the Master that is doing the attunement and unfortunately is another side of Reiki that is highly disturbing in its consequences. By using their own energy (ego) it can cause huge problems in the student's health and welfare, which in turn can manifest into a physical or mental illness.

The same can be said when they use their own energy for "healing" a client. By using your own energy, it will transfer all your negative thoughts and emotions to a totally unsuspecting client and will also leave you feeling drained and depleted.

Some Reiki Masters claim that we need to go into "trance" to allow Reiki to flow. Not true! Start putting obstacles in the way and it will stop the flow. Reiki is all about intent; you intend and Reiki flows, simple as.

As I explained earlier in the book, I was ridden with nerves when faced with my first Reiki healing and thought that I had to concentrate and try to aim the energy where Rapid River had shown me the problem. How naive was I, but like everything else in life, Reiki is a learning curve. The only difference is that we do not have to learn anything other than to be a divine and loving conduit for the Reiki energy to flow.

The more that you use Reiki, whether on yourself or others, the more you will get to know how it "feels"; your confidence will grow stronger and with confidence comes belief and with belief comes trust, which is all that is asked of us.

Trusting and becoming attuned to the Reiki energy is all that you need to do in order to change your way of life, enabling you to create a life beyond your wildest dreams.

Being attuned by a Reiki Master who has devoted their life to Reiki since they were first attuned is a must; a Reiki Master who is a clear and loving conduit, enabling you to be attuned with pure Divine Source Reiki energy. This will allow you to go forward and do what you have been sent here to do; heal and teach the ways of our Lord Jesus.

First and Second degree Reiki are specifically about "clearing" all negative thoughts, doubts and memories that you may have buried in your subconscious.

First Degree Reiki as it was first taught is for you and you alone, enabling all negative thoughts, desires and emotions to be brought to your conscious level of thinking, which in turn allows you to deal with them in a positive way.

Subconscious events and occurrences that have been "buried" can be brought forward when you are in a dream state or meditating when the mind is open to receiving. This is perfectly normal and is how it should be to get you to where you need to be by the time you are ready for attunement to Second Degree Reiki.

My attunement to Second Degree Reiki brought to the surface all the negative emotions that had occurred from the death of my mum. This was an extremely difficult time for me and I felt that I was reliving every painful minute all over again.

My grief at losing mum had to be cleared and brought to the surface so that I could become a clear and loving channel for Divine Source Reiki at Master level.

The Solar Plexus is where we store all of our emotions and if we do not "get rid" of them, this is when they can manifest into a physical illness. My emotions manifested into my gall bladder becoming inflamed and having to have it removed. The Solar Plexus is the place your hands immediately go to if you experience a shock. It is the ultimate "holder" of all our feelings and from where our "gut instinct" comes from.

Second Degree Reiki deals with our emotional and mental wellbeing and follows on from First Degree Reiki in helping us to delve deeper into our subconscious thoughts and emotions. Reiki 2 also opens additional energy centres allowing you to "connect" to a greater volume of Divine Source Reiki and to become a clear and loving conduit for the energy to flow through you without any kind of interference.

Once you have been attuned to these two Reiki degrees, you may feel that you want to go on to become a Reiki Master. The Usui System of Reiki is a way of life for its Masters and is to be treated with honour and respect with an appreciation for the simplicity and the undeniable power of Reiki.

It is up to you to honour your commitment to healing yourself and others and to promote the importance of tolerance and a non-aggressive way of life. Being a Reiki Master entails being a leader who has serious responsibilities that are not to be taken lightly, remembering also that you are still a student of Reiki.

As your life grows with Reiki, you never stop learning; and getting together with other people who are at a similar level of spiritual development will help you to achieve balance between your own individual development and theirs.

The next logical step is to become attuned to the Reiki Master/Teacher energy for those with the will and desire to teach Reiki.

Reiki Masters agree to use the form as it is, protected by the current lineage bearer Phyllis Lei Furumoto. Mrs Furomoto carries the seed of Usui Shiki Ryoho passed from one generation to another and for this, we as Reiki students must show the utmost respect.

Reiki as a way of life is about surrendering to the flow and guidance of the Reiki energy and becomes an exciting way to trust life without the need to know why.

Remember that Reiki is a "life choice" and you still have the free will to go in whatever direction you choose, but my advice is to allow Reiki to "choose" for you the life that is for your Highest and Greatest good!

> *We are not human beings having*
> *a spiritual experience;*
>
> *But spiritual beings having a human experience*
>
> ~ **Pierre** Teilhard de Chardin ~

Learning Non-Attachment

I am very often asked how I manage to stay "detached" from my clients, whether in Reiki or when I am counselling a bereaved client. My answer is that I have to be professional in the same way as, say, for a doctor or a lawyer. I cannot afford to take everyone's problems on board and, if that were the case, I would have nothing left to give.

How do I do it and still remain empathic? I honestly believe first and foremost that it is a gift that I have been given and, secondly, "grounding and protecting at all times".

Dr. Usui also learned from living in the beggar quarter of Kyoto the importance of non-attachment to the results of his healings. It is possible that some of the beggars needed to live out their lives in the beggars' quarter in order to learn certain lessons, so who are we to judge this as right or wrong?

In some ideology it is proclaimed that some human beings choose their own suffering or dis-ease as a means of redemption for mistakes made in the past.

To a gifted healer such as Usui, to try to interfere with a premature healing might be a real transgression into a person's essential life process. With this knowledge it became very clear to Usui that it was not his job to use his incredible gift to heal the world, but instead to show people how they might help to heal themselves first and foremost.

This same belief applies even today and even Jesus proclaimed that we are not the ones who decide who lives and who dies. That choice is ultimately left to the client who decides how much Reiki they wish to take or not, as the case may be.

To forgive is the highest, most beautiful form of love.

***In return, you will receive untold
peace and happiness***

*~ **Robert** Muller ~*

Reiki and Dying

Reiki can be used when someone is about to make their transition to the "other side", helping them to pass over with a reality of a continuing existence, less pain and emotional turmoil. Reiki can also help to comfort those who are left behind.

It is always best to explain this to your client and their families as their expectations may be unrealistic and will also help to clarify that we, as Reiki practitioners, do not perform miracles or promise cures. (This premise is also advisable when doing treatments on your clients).

Many people have found that having a Reiki treatment assists them in making the effort to find healing and gives them hope, whilst others find that Reiki helps them to accept the inevitable.

Reiki can be used with the intention that it makes the soul's transition easier, bringing solace to the bereaved and helping to eliminate any fear and anger. Reverence and respect for this process is extremely important and during this time it is imperative that the Practitioner remains grounded at all time.

Being a facilitator at the transition between life and death means that we are in effect, holding that person's spiritual hand as they make the transition out of their physical body into their Spiritual body.

A case in point was Gwen, whom I mentioned earlier in my book. Gwen had been diagnosed with terminal lung cancer and been given a matter of weeks to live. Remember how Jock, Gwen's husband, came forward during the healing with a personal message for her, so that when the time came for her own transition she passed over with a smile on her face?

Having the prior knowledge that Jock was going to be there waiting for Gwen, helped her family to cope, in however small a way, with such a monumental loss.

"Everyone dies, but no one is dead."

Ancient Tibetan saying

- Anon -

Working with the "Light"

Before we begin any kind of work where we are going to be "working with the light", we need to ground and protect our "aura", our own personal energy field and it is an essential part of our daily practice.

Grounding and protecting is so important to your spiritual development. As you start to become more attuned to the energy work, your light begins to burn brighter and therefore negative energy will try to latch on to this 'light' and drain you.

Following is a prime example: You have been to town/work/socialising and arrive home feeling totally drained and depleted. The simple reason why you feel this way is because everyone with whom have come into contact has taken a little bit of your "aura", leaving you feeling exhausted and devoid of all energy.

Very often these people are portrayed as psychic vampires, "bleeding" you of every last bit of "energy" that you have got. This happens on a subconscious level without you or the "taker" having any idea at what has occurred between you, hence the need to protect your aura at all times.

An explanation to why we must ground ourselves is to help us keep focused on every day matters and also helps to give us clarity of thought and vision. Grounding is a process that helps the body to connect to earth energies via its root chakra.

You can always tell when someone is not grounded. They are usually "away with the fairies" and cannot reasonably quantify their thoughts and actions. Because we are first and foremost spiritual beings, the physical body is sometimes neglected hence the importance of undertaking the following grounding and protection exercise. It is never too late to do this exercise if you happen to forget first thing in a morning. It will always be there for you and, just by putting the intent up, prayers will be answered.

Grounding

Imagine in your mind's eye, roots beginning to sprout from the soles of your feet and extending down into Mother Earth until you see in front of you a rock crystal. Taking note of the colour of the rock, you are aware that your roots are wrapping themselves around this crystal and firmly anchoring you to Mother Earth.

Protection

I want you to imagine a breast plate being placed over your shoulders reaching down to your waist and covering your Solar Plexus Chakra, back and front. You can now feel a huge cloak (Scottish widows) enfolding your body from shoulders to feet, with the hood coming up and over your head to just above your brow chakra (third eye).

If you wish, you may also ask the Divine Source/Angelic Realm for extra protection. Remember that this is free will and they will not interfere unless you invite them in.

You aura is now fully grounded and protected.

An exercise I use to show how the protection with the cloak and shield works is by using a pendulum and, standing in front of a student, I "ask" if it will work for me. If it starts to swing in a clockwise direction the answer is "yes" and will continue swinging in this manner even when you move further away from student.

This always shocks them when they realise how far their energy field goes out from the body and gives evidence that it can be walked through at a great distance.

When I ask them to "put" the shield and cloak back on, they are amazed to see that the pendulum stops working and for the simplest of reasons, because their energy field (aura) is now "under cover".

Every human being is the author of his own health or disease.

Buddha

Explanation of the Aura

The aura is the energy field that surrounds all living things and is totally unique to you as a living, breathing human being. Without this energy field, we would not exist; it is your very own blue print.

As I explained earlier, when working with the "White Light", your aura will start to "light" up like a Belisha beacon. That is why it is imperative that you protect your energy field every day before you start mixing with "Joe public".

Your aura can be flexible due to your emotions, state of health, energy levels and also your outlook on life. The aura can also be weakened by alcohol, drugs, stress, poor diet, lack of sleep and exercise. It is also a pointer to how you are feeling in yourself; it can also reflect your maturity, your health and moods with negative thoughts and emotions affecting the aura in a quite substantial way.

For example, you find yourself in someone's company and, without warning the hairs on your arms stand on end, making you feel really uncomfortable in their presence. The simple answer is that you are a "sensitive" and you are picking up on their negativity; your subconscious does not like what it is feeling, hence the prickles being sent out as a warning.

The aura is also a strong indicator of your spiritual and physical attributes. Overall, this remains the same, subject to major changes that may occur in your life and strongly reflecting both positive and negative thoughts.

Words were never invented to fully explain the peaceful aura that surrounds us when we are in communion with minds of the same thoughts

~ Eddie Myers ~

Descriptive Layers of the Aura/ Human Energy Field and Chakra locations.

- The **First Layer** of your aura is the **Physical Layer**. This is the basic magnetic field around the physical body

- The **Second Layer** is the **Etheric Layer**. Any disharmony, pain or disturbance can be felt or seen here. This is the layer that is commonly used when giving spiritual healing

- The **Third layer** is the **Vital Layer**, which will react to dynamic changes in thought patterns in the Etheric and Emotional layers

- The **Fourth Layer** is the **Emotional Layer**. This area will often show confusion, as thought patterns are forever changing by mental attitude. Both negative and positive vibrations are normally shown in this layer

- The **Fifth Layer** is the **Lower Mental Layer** and shows the development and growth that has taken place

- The **Sixth Layer** is the **Higher Mental Layer** relating to the soul and is part of the Universal Consciousness, shows the nearness to God, with the desire to follow and understand the belief within

- The **Seventh Layer** is the **Spiritual Layer** composed of pure light, the Spirit self. This layer is not seen by the human eye as it is pure light. By using Kirlian photography, the aura appears in more detail, very often as a halo surrounding the head. It is of fine energy and close to the cosmic consciousness

- Our aura is the energy that animates our physical body. Aura is life and without it we would simply not exist!

- Our physical bodies are surrounded by seven layers of the auric field and can be divided into two planes; **Physical and Spiritual**, **Etheric, Emotional and Mental** planes and, finally, the **Astral** body, which is the bridge between the physical and spiritual levels of our auric field

- The outer/higher layers of our aura consist of the **Etheric, Celestial** and **Ketheric** bodies

Each layer of the auric field is a body, just as real as the physical body. Each layer has its own sense of purpose, interconnecting with the others and determining our experience with our every day physical reality.

Your own personal energy system is conscious energy and connects with all energies that exist in the Universe; the physical, metaphysical and spiritual world.

Protecting your aura every day means that you are looking after your energy systems; the physical, emotional, intellectual and spiritual, which consist of your deepest and most profound needs.

Colours of the Aura

Below is a detailed explanation of the colours of the aura which in turn relates to the colour of the crystal that you see in the grounding exercise.

Red is filled with desire, vitality and the urge to win at all times. Craves success, loves sports, competing and is a natural born leader. Attributes to this colour include strength, courage, passion, eroticism, earthiness, practicality and a desire for possessions. Has a sense of adventure with a basic survival instinct.

Orange gives you the ability to reach out and extend yourself towards others. If you have this colour in your aura it usually points to a creative person who relates to others in an open and friendly manner. Sociable, intuitive, confident and trusts their "strong gut feelings".

Yellow denotes a sunny and enthusiastic person, a great sense of humour and a cheerful, optimistic outlook. Intellectual, open to new ideas, filled with happiness and warmth with the ability to relax at all times. Has a unique talent for organising people and places.

Green in your aura denotes tenacity, patience, perseverance, with high ideals and aspirations. Desiring respectability and personal attainment; puts a high value on work and career with adaptability.

Blue evokes very deep feelings, empathy and skill at communication. Attaches great importance to personal relationships with loyalty, trust, desire and devotion a priority and has a tendency to put the needs of others before their own. Likes to meditate, bit of a dreamer, enjoys solitude, emotionally sensitive and intuitive. Prefers a calm, peaceful tranquil environment at all times.

Violet connects with the higher consciousness and higher realms. Compassionate, has psychic abilities, sensitive and original in trying to make their dreams come true. Tries hard to be non-judgemental, appreciates kindness and compassion from other like minded souls, but with a tendency to be a bit of a dreamer.

White is the colour usually surrounding a Light Worker's aura. It is spiritually motivated and open and receptive to the Divine or spiritual world.

As your "connection" becomes stronger you will notice that your "colours" become brighter and more visible, allowing you to access what colour is right for you as you progress in your Spiritual development.

I liken an aura to a mirage that you see "shimmering" just above the surface of the ground on a hot summer's day. There are numerous ways of "seeing" the aura. The easiest one that I teach to my students is to go outside at night and "look" at the night sky. Keeping the image of the mirage in mind notice how trees, buildings, etc. seem to "glow" in the dark. This is the aura, energy field and surrounds every living thing here on Mother Earth.

Another easy exercise is to get someone to sit against a light coloured wall, preferably with dim lighting. Allow your eyes to become lazy and, looking beyond their head, you should see their outline start to "shimmer". The more that you practice, the easier it becomes and will, eventually, get to the stage where you will automatically see auras.

Spirit vibrates at a higher level of energy, which means that most of the population are not able to connect and this is where Reiki comes into being. Becoming attuned to Reiki will allow you access to a higher vibration and if you so wish, connection to the Spirit world.

As I stated earlier in my book, several of my clients have felt the need to know their deceased loved ones are still around. Having this contact gives a greater sense of peace and comfort and also helps them to come to terms with their sad loss, enabling them to live with their grief.

I can never promise to deliver, but having said that, "they" never fail to make contact. It's almost as if they were waiting for the moment when they could reconnect with their loved ones still "down here" on the Earth plane.

We also have to remember and respect that not everyone wants to make this connection and some would find it extremely uncomfortable and frightening.

My own belief on death and grief is that you never get over it, but you do learn to live with it. Everyone's grief is different and we have to respect that and allow everyone to grieve in their own way, however long it takes.

Come to me in my dreams, and then
By day I shall be well again!
For then the night will more than pay
The hopeless longing of the day!

- Matthew Arnold -

Explanation to Chakras:
Your Own Personal Energy System

Chakra is a Sanskrit word meaning wheel and it refers to the seven energy centres in our body. Chakras and their functions were first mentioned in the Vedas, which were ancient Hindu texts of knowledge.

Our chakras regulate the flow of energy, but are not physical. They are aspects of consciousness in the same way as our aura is an aspect of consciousness with the mind and the physical body working together. They work through the endocrine and nervous system in the physical body and are therefore associated with particular parts and organs of the body. Each sense, feeling and experience is divided into seven categories and is therefore allocated to a specific chakra.

When you feel stress in your consciousness, you feel it in the chakra associated with that part of your consciousness and in the part of the physical body where each individual chakra is located. This can lead to negative energy being "stored" in the relevant chakra, which in time could manifest into a physical/mental illness.

Everything can be healed, so in understanding the chakras the healing process can begin with the mind and the body. Chakras that are out of line and not "spinning" properly means that the physical, mental and emotional bodies are not working in harmony with one another so, enabling "illness" to manifest.

Stress is the biggest killer of all and is the main reason behind today's "modern illnesses". Using the pendulum to dowse and balance the chakras, bringing them back into line and spinning at the correct frequency, enables the client to release the stress causing the symptoms, which in turn creates a feeling of wellbeing.

Chakras are linkage points between your aura and the subtle bodies that form the "bio-magnetic" sheath around your physical body; each chakra links to a specific area of life and to various organs and conditions.

The chakras below the waist are primarily physical, where as those in the upper torso are aligned to emotional functioning that can create psychosomatic[3] conditions.

Chakras in the head function on a mental intuitive base, with the third eye and crown chakras functioning at a spiritual level where we connect to the Divine Source energy.

Chakras that are stuck open are known as "blown" and, because there is no protection, can also be open to negative influences. Likewise a chakra can be in a closed position, leading to blockages, allowing negative qualities to collect in this area, which ultimately leads to dis-ease manifesting in the physical body.

---

[3] Describes a physical illness that is caused by mental factors such as stress or the effects related to such illnesses.

By balancing the equilibrium (forces or factors) in all chakras, a physical state or sense of wellbeing will maintain a bodily balance. It is still possible to clear and balance a chakra after a physical illness has manifested itself there.

This was a case in point with Cheryl and how negative energy had become "stuck" in her lower chakras, leading to her suffering with suspected Endometriosis.

The same scenario could also be applied to Doreen, *Polly and *Sally.

My negative emotions from dealing with Mum's illnesses from the age of seven manifested into my Solar Plexus, culminating in the removal of my gallbladder in 1972, as mentioned earlier in the book.

Spheres and Colours of the Chakras

Below is a detailed explanation to the spheres and colours connecting to each relevant chakra- energy centre in the body!

Earth Chakra (beneath the feet): The sphere of everyday reality and grounding. Imbalances or blockages lead to discomfort in your physical body; feelings of helplessness and inability to function practically in the world.

Base Chakra (base of your spine/perineum);
The sphere of basic survival and security issues! Imbalances lead to sexual disturbances and feelings of anger, impotence and frustration.

Sacral Chakra (navel; slightly below waist): The sphere of creativity, fertility and acceptance of yourself as a sexual being. Imbalances lead to infertility and blocked creativity. The sacral chakra is where "hooks" from other people may be felt, particularly from sexual encounters.

Solar Plexus Chakra (just above waist): The sphere of emotional communication and assimilation. Blockages can lead to you taking on other people's feelings and problems, or to being overwhelmed by your own emotions. It affects energy assimilation and utilisation, leaving you feeling totally drained and depleted. Emotional "hooks" from other people can also be found here.

Heart Chakra (over heart): The sphere of love and nurturing. If your heart chakra is blocked, love cannot flourish. Feelings such as jealousy and resentment are common and there is enormous resistance to change.

Higher Heart Chakra (thymus gland - between the heart and throat): The sphere of compassion. If this chakra is blocked, unconditional love and service cannot be offered. You will be emotionally needy and unable to express your feelings openly.

Throat Chakra (centre of your throat): The sphere of communication. If this chakra is blocked, your thoughts and feelings cannot be verbalised. Other people's opinions may cause you difficulty.

Brow Chakra (third eye - above and between your eyebrows): The sphere of intention and mental connection. Imbalances can give you a feeling of being bombarded by other people's thoughts, or being overtaken by wild and irrational intuitions that have no basis in truth. Controlling or coercing mental "hooks" from other people can lock in here and affect your thoughts.

Crown Chakra (top of head): The sphere of spiritual communication and awareness;

If the crown chakra is blocked, attempting to control others is common. If this chakra is "stuck open", obsession and openness to spiritual interference or possession can result.

Higher Crown Chakra (above your head): The sphere of service and spiritual enlightenment. If this chakra is "stuck open", you are spaced out and open to delusion. Influence from other realms of beings and entity are liable to become attached.

Spleen Chakra (below left armpit): The sphere of association and empowerment. If this chakra is imbalanced, you will have anger issues or suffer constant irritation with your body turning in to attack itself. If the chakra is too open, other people can draw on your energy leaving you depleted, particularly at the immune level.

Past Life Chakra (Three fingers' breadth behind your ears, just above bony ridge): The sphere of memory and hereditary issues. Imbalances mean that you are stuck in the past and cannot move forward and may well be repeating your own past life/ancestral patterns that have passed down through your family. This is also the point where people from your past can attach and control you.

Emotion always has its roots in the unconscious and manifests itself in the body!

-Irene Claremont de Castillejo -

Explanation and Sanskrit Name of Each Individual Chakra

Below is an explanation to each individual body part linked to its own Chakra and the problems that can arise in the physical body when one becomes blocked with negative energy.

Each chakra has its own Sanskrit name and image.

Muladhara; Base Chakra: Located at the base of the spine. Body parts associated: spine, legs, feet, skeletal system, large intestine, kidneys and adrenal glands. Malfunction can cause sciatica, constipation, haemorrhoids and obesity.

Svadisthana; Sacral Plexus or Spleen Chakra: Located above the pubic bone. Body parts associated: bladder, kidneys, spleen, and womb, reproductive and circulatory systems.

Malfunction can cause uterine, bladder, kidney and impotence problems.

Manipuri; Solar Plexus: Located in the midriff. Body parts associated; stomach, gall bladder, pancreas, small intestine, digestive and nervous system. Malfunction can cause diabetes, ulcers and eating disorders, to name but a few.

Anahata; Heart Chakra: Located in middle of the chest. This chakra relates to the heart, lungs, thymus and circulatory glands. Malfunction can cause heart and lung disease, asthma and blood pressure, to name but a few.

Vishuddi; Throat Chakra: Located in the throat. Body parts associated: thyroid, parathyroid, throat, mouth, neck and hypothalamus. Malfunction can cause sore throat, swollen glands, thyroid and speech problems.

Ajna; **Brow or Third Eye:** Located just above bridge of nose. Body parts associated: brain, eyes, ears, nose, pituitary and pineal glands. Malfunction can cause migraine, nightmares, poor concentration and vision problems.

Saharara; Crown Chakra: Located on top of head. Body parts associated: pineal gland, cerebral cortex and the central nervous system. The Crown Chakra is where Divine Source energy is channelled through you to your client, allowing them to use this energy for self healing. (Remember, it is the client who is the "healer" and will only take as much Reiki as their subconscious needs).

The above information is just a rough guideline to what can manifest when each individual chakra is blocked and, hopefully, you have a better idea of each chakra's role in energy exchange between your body and the world around you.

It is important to realise that by balancing your chakras it will help to resolve physical, emotional and spiritual issues and means your entire body will begin to resonate and give off slightly higher frequencies than before. This can often be felt as a sense of relief.

Yet this is health: To have a body functioning so perfectly that when its few simple needs are met it never calls attention to its own existence.

- Bertha Stuart Dyment -

The Angelic Realm

St. Thomas Aquinas said, "Angels transcend every religion, every philosophy and creed. In fact, Angels have no religion as we know it. Their existence precedes every religious system that has ever existed on Earth."

The word Angel is derived from the Greek word "Angelos" and means "messenger". Jesus himself declared that angels are not dead saints or holy people living on the earth and most people have a vague idea of what an Angel is, but to others they are a total fabrication of the imagination, fairy tale characters even.

They are part of God's creation and my own personal belief is that Angels are aspects of the Divine Source of all ONE.

I am often asked what "God" is and my answer is always the same. To me God is a "Higher Energy" that we can all call on in our hour of need. This energy is neither male nor female, just "ALL THAT IS" and is there for everyone, irrespective of race, creed or colour.

God created the Angels as a totally different species from humankind. Humans can never become angels, but those of us that walked with Jesus two centuries ago have now reincarnated as Earth Angels; Light Workers with a propensity to love our fellow man and to try and teach the beliefs of our Master, Jesus.

The Angels represent God's loving care for us and also serve God's purpose in helping us to "find" our way in life. Each individual Angel has a specific role in helping us in the way that we need to be helped. Just as we ask for help from professionals who provide us with specific skills and expertise, each individual Angel has their own special skill in the Angelic Realm.

With practice and especially meditation you can connect to the Angel that is specific to your needs, allowing them to assist with whatever you need to be helped with at any given time. They also want you to know that you are never alone!

Angels love to interact with every aspect of life, but they cannot do that unless you specifically ask them to and this is where "Free Will" comes into being. To ask (free will) for their assistance, all you have to say is, "Angels, please help me," and simply by you invoking the request for help, they will be at your side immediately.

All you have to do then is to listen to that little voice inside your head and also to go with what your gut instinct is "telling" you.

These examples are the ways that the Angels step into our lives and help to guide us to where we need to be to enrich and fulfil our lives to the maximum. It is when we do not "listen" to what our gut instinct/voices are screaming at us that life becomes a constant battle.

People who have suffered from negative experiences such as a traumatic, abusive upbringing, or ridicule from "friends", workmates, etc. find it hard to believe there is such a thing as a God or Angels.

A prime example is Bryn, who I met on holiday in Egypt. As I explained to him, God and the Angels know how you feel and they want to help you regain the joy of knowing and experiencing a loving God; a God who understands all your hurt and pain. Just by giving all these negative emotions over to him and the Angelic Realm you will be amazed at how your thoughts and feelings will become more heart centred and loving.

However minute you think the problem may be to you, God and the Angelic Realm will always be there ready to help. Trust is the key word; trusting in God and the Angels will bring you a life that is full of satisfaction with a happiness that knows no bounds.

You know that "gut" feeling that you get deep down in the pit of your stomach (solar plexus) when all your basic instincts are screaming out at you that something is not quite right, but you decide to ignore it? This is when life becomes extremely difficult; life's aims become unachievable, leaving you feeling a total failure at everything that you try to do.

I speak from experience when I say that I chose to ignore what my gut instinct kept telling me and the outcome for me was to end up both physically and mentally exhausted, and all because I did not listen to what I was being "told".

Nevertheless, we are all human and think we know best.

I had to become very ill with reactive stress and depression before I finished work voluntarily. The outcome from doing what the Angels had asked me to do, is for me now to be living my life's purpose; Reiki. Simple as that!

Angels can fly because they take themselves lightly

~ G.K. Chesterton ~

An Explanation of Archangels

All Archangels' names end with the "el" suffix, which means "in God". The first half of the name symbolises the speciality of each individual Angel.

Angels/Archangels are able to be in many places at any one given time.

The most prominent Archangels to which the majority of us can all relate are Michael, Raphael, Gabriel, Uriel, Sandalphon and Metatron.

- **Archangel Michael** is there to protect and guide in all aspects of your life
- **Archangel Raphael** supervises healers and healing for all of Earth's population
- **Archangel Gabriel** is known as the "messenger" Angel. Gabriel means, "God is my strength" and is a teacher and messenger of truth
- **Archangel Uriel** means the "Light of God" and helps to bring peace, stability and determination into our lives

- **Archangel Sandalphon** is known as the Angel of Mercy and Prayer and is also the Archangel that rules the seventh heaven and was known as the Prophet Elijah when he was on the Earth plane

 After being transported to heaven in a burning chariot and whilst still alive, Elijah became Archangel Sandalphon in order to be of service to God. He holds a position in the angelic hierarchy behind **Merkabah - The Heavenly chariot!** **Sandalphon** is said to the tallest of all the Angels, reaching easily from Earth to the Heavens, allowing him to "whisper" in God's ear.

 Sandalphon is charged with anchoring the Light onto Earth, and will assist Lightworkers to do the same, both into the planet and into our own energy bodies. He said "I am an anchor. I act to penetrate a body and anchor myself into it as a conduit of Light energy, keeping things working at root level in accordance with the Divine Plan, whilst simultaneously channelling in Divine Light, supplying all that is required in order for balance, harmony and hence stability to be achieved."

Archangel Sandalphon appeared to me in answer to prayers concerning my friend, Paul Thomas. A "huge" golden figure with wings suddenly appeared in the corner of my bedroom, reaching from floor to ceiling. He introduced himself as Archangel Sandalphon and told me he had come in answer to my prayers concerning Paul.

He was to give me a deeply profound message for Paul and is a "constant" whenever he needs him.

He was also to appear to my friend *Jackie in answer to her pleas for her son-in law and his family. Whilst channelling a healing for Jackie, she was to "see" this bright golden "Angel" standing in front of her when on her "Sacred Reiki Journey".

I showed her a picture of Archangel Sandalphon and she immediately confirmed that that was who she had "seen". Jackie was to "ask" him for help regarding her son-in-law's job prospects.

*Mark had been made redundant a few months before and was getting really despondent about finding work. Being a father of three children and with a wife to support, things were getting really tough. That was on the Thursday. The following Monday Mark received a phone call inviting him to attend an interview that afternoon, following which he was offered the job!

To call upon Archangel Sandalphon with an urgent prayer that you need answered, say the following words and insert your prayer regarding your desire:

"Beloved Archangel Sandalphon, deliverer and answerer of all prayers. I, (your name) ask for your assistance now. Please deliver my prayer (insert prayer) to God as soon as possible. I ask that you relay a clear message to me that will I easily understand. Please update me as to the progress of my request and let me know if I need to do anything else.
Thank you,
Namaste and Amen"

His twin brother, Archangel Metatron, known as the Prophet Enoch when he walked the earth, is also known as the "Chancellor of Heaven" and in folklore is rumoured to be more powerful than Michael or Gabriel and holds the link between human and the divine.

The name Metatron means "One who occupies the throne next to the throne of the Divine". He is also known as the Patron Angel of Children and is the only Angel without the suffix "El".

Metatron was the Angel that led the children of Israel through the wilderness to safety and continues to lead children today, both on earth and in heaven.

Archangel Metatron has a special place in his heart for children, especially those who are spiritually gifted and the new Indigo, Rainbow and Crystal Children are under his Angelic guidance.

This generation of psychically sensitive children have ongoing problems related to allergies, misdiagnoses, fitting in and questioning abuse of authority.

My own daughter Cheryl is an Indigo and all the above she has had to cope with during this lifetime.

Archangel Metatron, acutely aware of the Indigo and Crystal children's needs, can help you as a parent or teacher; in fact, anyone who is involved in raising or teaching these very special and wise souls.

Doreen Virtue's "The Care and Feeding of Indigo Children" and "The Crystal Children" are very informative books for those parents with "special" children and help's to understand and cope with their needs.

Archangel Metatron will help you connect to your own truth and higher self just by asking. He also helps to keep our minds and thoughts free of clutter, so that we are ready and able to receive the truths that will allow us to become the best we can be.

Archangels are the divination aspects of God's love for us and we can learn to trust their assistance and to accept their guidance without fear of being let down.

Angels know our every thought, deed, word and action. Each and every one of you has an Angel walking beside you, ready and waiting for you to invite them to help with any problems that you may have and which needs urgent "attention".

All that is required is for you to place all of your problems, however big or small, into their loving hands and let them work for your highest and greatest good; in other words, what is good and best for you.

Sitting back and expecting the world to come to you is not about giving your life over to the Angelic Realm. By "listening" and going with your "gut instinct", you allow yourself to be guided by these Angelic beings and henceforth life can only get better.

Once we have made this conscious decision of allowing the Angels to step in and help, we can then witness what doors are opening and what doors are closing, allowing us to move forward confidently and with a feeling of positivity that it is right for us.

Angels are always with us and eager to help. They are loving and supportive partners in all of our endeavours. They help us to reach beyond our fears to our highest and best expressions of ourselves. This is a powerful way of practising the wisdom of "letting go and letting God". Not an easy thing to do, but with practice it becomes simple, almost like second nature. Trust and let go!

The Angels' assistance is available to us whenever or wherever we are. Simply by asking for their help, they will be at your side immediately.

You may question why I am so certain in my beliefs and my answer is simple: I have been helping people connect more deeply with their Angels for help and assistance for some time now and I also speak from my own experiences. The testimonials at the back of the book confirm the positive outcomes that come about through letting these celestial beings into your life!

We all know that Angels are truly universal and are fundamental to all of the world's major religions. We find them in Christianity, Islam, Judaism, Buddhism and Hinduism, ranging from the Middle East to the West, from the Old to the New Testament and from the Vedas[4] to the Koran.

It tells in the Bible of Archangel Gabriel bringing the Annunciation that Jesus will come to Mary; Luke 1:26–37 (MKJV)

In Islamic tradition, Archangel Gabriel is renowned for dictating the Holy Koran to the Prophet Mohammed.

The Angelic annunciations show us that whatever religion, creed or doctrine we follow, Angels are universal and are there for us all to share. They are not judgemental as we are, do not make fun of someone who is just that little bit different to what we as a society regard as "normal".

We are just mere mortals and should be assisting our fellow man in a helpful and loving way.

The Angels love each and every one of us unconditionally. They are a universal human experience. They bring messages from a higher order of loving consciousness to us; Divine Angelic messages that help us to realise that we are not alone, that we need not be afraid and assisting our ability to help one another.

We all need to listen and heed these words; to have a world where there are no wars, where man no longer feels he needs to kill and maim innocent people in the name of religion, a world where we can all love one God, whatever name he comes under, and to abide by his wishes to love and respect one another's beliefs as if it is our own flesh and blood.

---

4   Vedas; Hindu sacred texts originally transmitted orally, but written down in sacred books from the 6th century BC!

The Angels are here to help us and is their only reason for being. God created the Angels to care for mankind, bringing the same message to all cultures, and divides. Amen!

**Ask and it will be given to you;
seek and you will find.**

Knock and it will be opened to you

- Matthew 7:7 -

Testimonials to Belief and Believing!

Below are two emails from a lady that sits in my Reiki Circle and is now a personal friend. I have been working with Chris for the last few months on how the Angels, if allowed, can bring so many benefits into your life.

I attuned Chris to First Degree Reiki in January 2009, Second Degree Reiki in February 2010 and she is now opening up to the fact that the Angels that are there for everyone and that all you have to do is, ASK!

05 January 2010 13:53:27

This morning, I trundled' round to my garage, dropped some rubbish in the bin, got the car out of the garage, locked the garage up and drove into town. When I got to the town -end of Burton Road, I realised I hadn't picked up my handbag and put it in the car before I drove off. Needless to say, I sped back home, obviously worried about the consequences of some person walking off with my purse, cards, keys, etc. Having made a plea for help from the Angels earlier on, I was thinking that it had all been a waste of time, but of course when I got back home and my handbag was still where I had left it, untouched, I realised I had been completely wrong;, they had been there for me all the time and I had to apologise profusely for doubting them.

When will I learn, Maggie?
Chris xxx

Two days later and again they were showing Chris that "they" are near.

07 January 2010 16:06:04

They're with me again, Maggie.
Popped out at lunch time and some while after I got back I realised I was no longer wearing a fine gold wedding ring. I'd been to the Bank whilst I was out and had taken my gloves off there. I checked my gloves – nothing, I walked around the office – nothing.
Decided to ring the Bank – nothing
Then I remembered I'd washed my hands – went to our toilets, emptied the bin of all the damp paper towels and there it was nestling in the bottom of the bin.
An hour later and the cleaners would have emptied the bin and that would have been that.
What can I say?
Chris xxx

Just because it's not what you were expecting, doesn't mean it's not everything you've been waiting for...

- Unknown -

25 January 2009

The day after Chris was attuned to First Degree Reiki, I received this message from her:

Yesterday two strange things happened to me, Maggie.

The first was (cutting a long story short), I've had a plant plot on my kitchen window sill for about four months where I was trying to grow several shrub cuttings, but despite some care (OK so they didn't get watered enough!), it was clear they weren't going to survive.

However, about two months ago, I noticed something was growing, so I left it so see what was happening. Sometime before the cuttings, I had planted a corm in the pot, but that had gone rotten and I'd given up, so I thought perhaps it was that coming to life after all.

Then the leaves grew and it looked like it could be a crocus, which I immediately discounted because I've never bought a crocus bulb in my life.

Yesterday when I got up, I there was a beautiful purple crocus in full bloom! Where did that come from? I've no idea, but I've taken it as a sign Reiki is for me.

Chris x

Twelve months on and Chris is now opening up to the inevitable; Reiki plus Angels is one powerful combination.

Grounding and Protecting Exercise
Bringing about Positive Results

*Celia was having problems at work and after showing her how to ground and protect herself, this was her email to me the following morning;

Good morning my lovely, what a good night and I have taken the strength and support from the circle and am surrounded by protection. I walked into the office this morning and felt strong and supported and just smiled. It works. Am actually buzzing inside is that normal!!

Love and light to you and I ask for strength for you to continue what you are doing. Bless you. I know you will say you are just a channel, but you and I both know what you have experienced in the past makes you who you are today.

I have to bless all those who have tried to make me fall because I pick myself up and go on.
YEAH!!
Celia xx

The following email from *Bryn touched me deeply:

15 July 2009 19:06:27

Dearest Mags & Pip,
I must admit Egypt had an effect on me. I think it helped me to consolidate my outlook on life and also to look at my inner self.
I spoke to my sister, Gwen, about the Reiki you performed on me and she was very impressed.

My feet are the best they have been for a long time; I don't know if this is due to the revising of my diet or the course of exercises that the Physio suggested that I do each day, or maybe it was the Reiki.
Whatever it is I'm pleased to be pain free.
Regards *Bryn & *Ali x

Helping Bryn to look at his inner self, consolidating his life for the better and bringing about this monumental change is beyond anything that I could ever express in words of gratitude; gratitude at being given the gift of reaching out to people and by example showing them what is out there for the taking.

From Eileen, my Reiki Student in Italy

Dear Mags,
Saturday 6th December was the first day of my new life and it's all thanks to my Reiki Master and Teacher - Margaret.
On this day, Margaret attuned me to Reiki 1 and I haven't looked back since.
She is so passionate about what she believes in that you can't help but be inspired.
Over a cup of tea before the lesson, we talked about spirituality, 'coincidences', angels – at last I felt a sense of belonging.
It was so nice to be able to talk with someone who understood how you felt about life, like never feeling as though you 'fitted in' or believing that there was something more but not quite sure what.
Margaret has since attuned me to Reiki 2 and although I believe she is a truly inspirational Reiki Master and Teacher,

she is, more importantly for me, a very sensitive person who cares deeply for all things.

She has helped me not only spiritually but also personally, giving in abundance the most precious gift we have – time.

I feel honoured that she calls me her friend.
Namaste
Eileen...x
Ps. I feel as though I can't leave without acknowledging her wonderful husband Pip. Together they really are a lovely couple. Cheers Pip!

From Lynn, who sits in Reiki Circle

Dear Margaret,
You have helped to turn my life around. Your kind words and wisdom have helped me see clearly on my darkest days. I came to see you feeling so low and desperate and your gentle kindness lifted me from the deepest, darkest hole I was in.

When I met Margaret, her smile lit up the room. She is a very caring and loving person who has lightened up my life. She is a great teacher, down to earth, very supportive and strict when we need it!

Margaret amazes me with her ability to stay positive, her strong faith in the higher self and her energy. At our first circle Margaret described her past experiences and her purpose in life. This resonated within me and I felt that, at last, I had met a kindred sole.

I truly believe that our small group has been a God send.
It is the one place where I feel totally accepted and held in love and respect.
Margaret? A true Earth Angel!
Love and light,
Lynn

From Rosie

Margaret is not Margaret; she is Margie-Mum to me! Meeting Margie-Mum was destiny and I am glad for the gift of having her in my life.

Margie-Mum has helped me to understand who I am and not to fight it but channel it in a way that is good for me as well as everyone else. She has been there when I needed it, even when I didn't realise myself that I did.

She is someone very special all wrapped inside a person who appears just like everyone else in order that those that need her can accept her and take what she has to give to them. No sandals, flowery kaftans and incense burning, but calm, kind, sensible Margie-Mum with a profound gift used with care and love.

Margie-Mum is a thoroughly modern Angel walking this earth and shining her light wherever it is needed.

Margie-Mum has had an interesting, challenging journey thus far and I am sure there are more adventures to be had along the way as she traverses her destined path.

It is an honour and a privilege to say Margie-Mum is a true and wonderful friend.

I look forward to saying one day, "See that lady on the TV, I know her and hope you get to know her too", as she travels the world receiving, giving & sharing in the light.

I hope that she receives as much love along the way as she dishes out!

Lotsa Luv,
Rosie x

At times our own light goes out and is rekindled by a spark from another person.

Each of us has cause to think with deep gratitude of those who have lighted the flame within us.

~ Albert Schweitzer ~

Being Attuned to First Degree Reiki

Rachel was first attuned to Reiki 1 in October 2008 and then came back to do Reiki 2 alongside Eileen in February 2009. She writes as follows:

Yet another wonderful, interesting and insightful day spent with Margaret and Eileen. Margaret is a competent and patient teacher and 'teaches' Reiki in an extremely approachable and enjoyable manner and I cannot recommend her highly enough.

So how has my life changed in the last few weeks since being attuned to Reiki 2?

The past few months after my Reiki 1 attunement, I have been troubled by anxiety attacks, which have at times been quite debilitating. I have felt confused and concerned about my future and felt quite sure that I would never feel truly 'happy' again.

I am pleased to say, that this has changed quite dramatically and for the better, and I am sure this is to do with my attunement to Reiki 2. A couple of days after my second attunement, I started to experience the vivid dreams again, the same as happened after my attunement to Reiki 1.

This time they weren't so upsetting, but again, I felt as though it was my subconscious clearing itself of some of my 'baggage'.

Over the period of the last few weeks I have noticed a distinct change in my demeanour. I have become more positive, more hopeful and, dare I say, much happier within myself.

I guess you could call this a sense of peace at times. My life just seems to be getting better.

I offer my thanks and blessings to the Greater Good and to Margaret, as without them both I would not be where I am today.

Love and light,
Rachel xxx

This email goes someway to justifying what I have already told you about how "Reiki" can "better" your life.

When I receive such a positive feedback like this one from Rachel, verifying that she has acknowledged the benefits of Reiki for her own Highest and Greatest good, a feeling of satisfaction resonates deep within; Namaste!

This next message is from Jackie, a lady that has come back into my life after many years apart. Jackie has had to tread a very difficult road in life thus far, including a difficult upbringing, the unexpected death of her first husband and a debilitating condition which she handles with much fortitude and humour and the occasional swear word!

Jackie also connected with Archangel Sandalphon, as explained earlier in this book.

Hi Mags,
What benefits have you brought into my life?
I perceive you as a kind caring person who always has time to listen to others.

It is obvious from talking to you for just a few minutes that you are a spiritual person and can share your perspective on life's events with others.

I also feel you have a way of telling it like it is in a way that people can accept.

You are a friend who is always there and ready to listen.

I can have deep conversations with you and am not afraid to talk about emotions or sensitive subjects.

I have become more in touch with my spiritual side and through you have regular contact with a circle of likeminded people.

I have learned about Reiki and healing and have confidence to use it myself.

I have gained knowledge of the need for grounding and protection and now use it in my daily routine.

Neighbours who usually ignore me have started being friendly.

Lovely lady in the Post Office carried a parcel to the car for me.

Found a white feather in my car!!

Had long conversation with lady at gym who said it was lovely to meet me and wanted to know my name (Big Head).

O2 have given me 40 free texts each month for the next three months.

I have recognised the benefits of positive thinking and now use this in my daily life.

Hope this e mail is not too boring.
Namaste,
Jackie xx

Distant Healing Reiki

I sent distant healing Reiki to Rachel who was suffering with a swollen abscess on her wisdom tooth.

Hi Mags,
Just wanted to say a HUGE thank you for the Reiki today... it's really helped! Within 10 minutes of me concentrating on you sending me healing, the constant throb in my tooth had gone to a dull ache and is now nearly gone. My mouth is still very tender and I can't bite down yet and also the side of my face is a little swollen...but the pain isn't half as bad as it was!
Thank you again!!!!
Lots of love and light,
Rach xxxxxx

From my very own Earth Angel; Wendy Joy Terry!

I consider my life to be truly blessed and I am filled with gratitude to have Margaret in my life. She is an extraordinary person so filled with pure love that her light simply flows from her.

Margaret is totally humbled to be in service of the Divine Source and is here on earth to do his will and help others on their pathway.

I thank Margaret for her tireless support and belief in me.

You make the world a better place!
Wendy Joy Terry
- Angel Teacher - Reiki first degree

> *The mind can assert anything and pretend it has proved it. My beliefs I test on my body, on my intuitional consciousness, and when I get a response there then I accept.*
>
> ~ D.H. Lawrence ~

I received the following email from Maja Milosavljević, who lives in Serbia formerly known as Yugoslavia. We became friends through her website listed below.

Dearest (((Mags))))xoxoxo,

I've read the Prologue of your book that you sent me, and I was overwhelmed with the intensity of the message; you've done such a wonderful job so far! It is absolutely gripping and I felt I was with you all those years...I've cried reading about your mom and how difficult it was for you to cope. You're so empathic yourself, and yes, an Earth Angel if there ever was one! This is so strongly channelled; your words are very profound and touching, yet your style is light and easy to read. I am so honoured you've shared it with me. I am so proud to be your friend!

The part where you talk about Amazing Grace - it was end of April-beginning of May 1972! At that moment here in ex-Yugoslavia, there was a terrible epidemic of Variola Vera, a deadly type of measles. My mom was due with me anytime and all hospitals were quarantined. Yet she left from the small town where they lived to capital Belgrade. Against all odds, and no vaccine taken, breaking through the military barricades, my mom came to Belgrade, determined that her baby would NOT die and had to be born in a hospital. She said she was guided by an unknown force, and she managed to give birth to me - May 5th, 1972, about the time Amazing Grace saved your life!!!

I guess my life was saved by an Amazing Grace too and we were destined to meet, you and I!

I absolutely LOVE what I've read so far and I know I'll love the whole book! I can't wait for it to be finished.

Thank you for letting me read it; I am blessed, honoured and very much obliged to you for your kindness and beautiful heart you shared here with me and will share with the world!

I love you dear soul sister!

Maja xx

http//www.thesmilingsoul.com

Epilogue

To wake up every morning and find Pip at my side makes me feel exceptionally loved in every way possible. I count my blessings and say "thank you" every day.

We have had nearly 35 years of marriage. My mum and dad had 31¼. Mum died at 59; I am still going strong at 63, four year longer than mum.

Whilst writing this book I have been having this recurring thought; did mum choose to suffer as she did to make me what I am today? Cheryl has also said that she knows she met nanny before she was born, even to telling me about the brown spots mum had on her left hand. Answer that one!

I am confident in the belief that Cheryl chose us as her parents, her being an Indigo child and also for her to help put me where I needed to be. Grahame is Grahame and dismisses everything that I stand for. I have no problem with that and refuse to argue the point with him. All will be revealed to him and the other doubters in this world in their own good time.

Saskatchewan/Rapid River; my dad! The more that I have traversed on this pathway, the more I am convinced that my Spirit guide, Saskatchewan is Dad, who has come back to assist and guide me in my Spiritual pathway.

(Whilst at the Spiritualist church, a psychic artist drew a picture of my guide as we were sitting in circle and the likeness to my dad was uncanny!)

I have recalled events that happened in my life that I had long forgotten about. But, I am steadfast in my belief that "they" wanted me to write a book detailing my life and to tell the world about Reiki, Divine Source and the Angelic Realm and, hopefully, I have achieved that with "their" help.

To be thrown upon one's own resources, is to be cast into the very lap of fortune;

For our faculties then undergo a development and display an energy of which they were previously unsusceptible

- Benjamin Franklin -

Amazing Grace:

Last but not least, an unexpected phone call:

2010 7 January 2010 at 19.15pm

I answered the phone and a voice said, "I hear that you have been searching for me; my name is Cynthia and I am "Amazing Grace" from your stay in hospital."

I was shocked, speechless and could not believe that at long last I was going to be speaking to the woman that I credit with saving my life; Amazing Grace, aka, Cynthia Hales, who is now a Rev Dr of Ministry and Divination.

What a start to 2010! I was beside myself with joy and excitement that at long last I was going to meet "Amazing Grace" and thank her for saving my life all those years ago.... my prayers had surely been answered!

*"Amazing Grace, how sweet the sound,
that saved a wretch like me....*

*I once was lost but now am found,
was blind, but now, I see.*

*T'was Grace that taught...my heart to
fear, and Grace, my fears relieved.*

*How precious did that Grace appear,
the hour I first believed!*

~ John Newton (1725–1807) ~

*We will meet again my friend,
A hundred years from today
Far away from where we lived
And where we used to play
We will know each others' eyes
And wonder where we met
Your laugh will sound familiar
Your heart, I won't forget
We will meet, I'm sure of this,
But let's not wait till then...
Let's take a walk beneath the stars
And share this world again.*

~ Ron Atchison ~

*Jesus Christ the same yesterday,
and today, and forever*

About the Author

Margaret Ann Elson is a Reiki Master at Teacher level.

Her Spiritual name is "Wise Owl" in recognition of her abilities as a Spiritual teacher.

Margaret has faced many difficulties in this lifetime, but the lessons she has learnt are to be shared in this book so that other Light Workers/ Earth Angels may find their true destiny in the not too distant future.

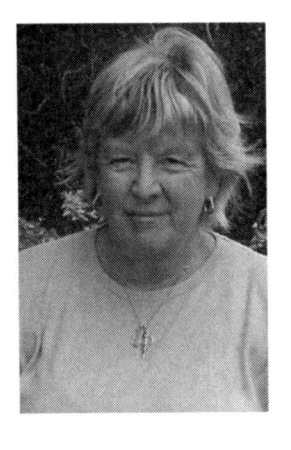

This book is a wakeup call for those souls amongst us who have not yet realised why they are here and to who they really are!